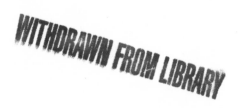

Lady Dragon

D·O·W·N SYNDROME

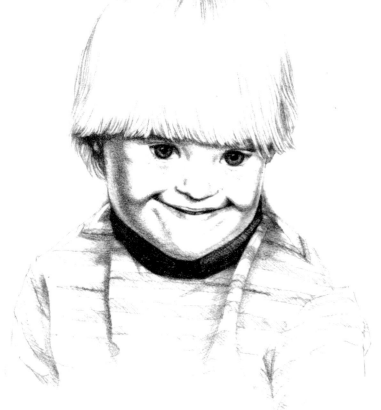

A Resource Handbook

CAROL TINGEY

DOWN SYNDROME

DOWN SYNDROME

A RESOURCE HANDBOOK

Edited by

Carol Tingey, Ph.D., F.A.A.M.D.
Early Intervention Research Institute
Utah State University
Logan, Utah

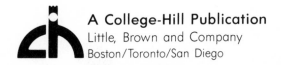

A College-Hill Publication
Little, Brown and Company
Boston/Toronto/San Diego

AA U 9 I 50

Illustrations by Elaine Sorenson.

College-Hill Press
A Division of
Little, Brown and Company (Inc.)
34 Beacon Street
Boston, Massachusetts 02108

Library of Congress Cataloging in Publication Data
Main entry under title:

Down syndrome.

- "A College-Hill publication."
Includes bibliographies and index.
1. Down's syndrome. 2. Down's syndrome—Patients—Family relationships.
I. Tingey, Carol, 1933- . [DNLM: 1. Down's Syndrome—handbooks.
WS 39 D748]
RJ506.D68D665   1988   618.92'858842   87-22526

ISBN 0-316-84562-0

Printed in the United States of America

CONTENTS

PREFACE

The telephone in my office rings often. Many of the calls are routine business, but sometimes there is a quiet, almost hesitant voice on the line. When I hear that voice, I lean back in my chair, take a deep breath, and, if I've worn uncomfortable shoes that day, slip off my shoes. The theme of the call will be something along this line: "They" gave me your name, and either I have a new baby with Down syndrome, or my brother/sister/ friend/son/daughter/neighbor has a new baby with Down syndrome. Other calls come from early intervention projects, special education teachers, group home parents, social workers, and psychologists. There are also the times when someone with the same story knocks unexpectedly at my office door.

It seems that for each of these people—parent, professional, friend— there are so many things that they suddenly need to know it is as if Down syndrome is an entirely new phenomenon on the day they first meet it. And so the questions begin.

Regardless of who is asking the questions, though, it is startling how similar they are. They center around two general themes that are not unusual in anyone's life. The first is about health and medical needs, and the second is about daily life and growing up. People want to know what special problems this person with Down syndrome might have. They want to know what to expect and how to enhance those expectations. And they want to know how the special needs of the person with Down syndrome might affect the lives of others.

The answers to these questions are seldom "yes" or "no," but are more often "if this, then that." And as I have listened and talked and talked and listened to these people—many of whom I will only meet over the phone—the stories I hear are about life and love. As the conversation progresses, and the minutes slip by, and especially if I need to hurry to a meeting, or write a report, or, if it is late Friday afternoon, to pick up my son, Jim (Jim has Down syndrome and is now 31, living in a group home. He left my home at 22, as his brothers and sister did. He and I have a date each Friday at five) I have wished over and over again that I had more time to share with each new contact all that I have learned about Down syndrome, from Jim and from all the other experts on Down syndrome whom I have been fortunate enough to meet. Realistically, I know that there will never be enough time, so I am pleased to have been able to organize the questions and to have answers ready, because I know that even if all the questions are answered today, there will be more people asking the same questions tomorrow.

I have been fortunate over the years to have had an opportunity to meet, study with, and get to know personally most of the people who have written about, researched, and worked with people who have Down syndrome. I have organized the questions I am asked into four sections—medical issues, family concerns, early development, and education and community activities—and I have asked those who know the most about these areas to share their wisdom in words that any of us can understand. The result is this book; the best answers from the most experienced people, almost the way you would hear it if you were talking with them yourself.

I am grateful to my professional friends for being willing to share their knowledge and experience, and for crowding yet another project into already overwhelming schedules, and to Elaine Sorenson for creating such delightful composite drawings of some of my personal friends who just happen to have Down syndrome. I also appreciate Vickie Richins, not only for the way she handles my busy telephone, but for her careful work with this manuscript and her generous attention to important details related to other work that needed to be done simultaneously. And thanks also to Debbie Risk for continuing to perform those services.

Carol Tingey
Logan, Utah

CONTRIBUTORS

Trish Boswell, B.S.
Teacher,
Granite School District,
Salt Lake City, Utah

John C. Carey, M.D., M.P.H.
Associate Professor, Pediatrics,
University of Utah,
Salt Lake City, Utah

Glendon Casto, Ph.D.
Director,
Early Intervention Research
  Institute,
Utah State University,
Logan, Utah

Diane Crutcher, M.S.
Executive Director,
National Down Syndrome
  Congress,
Park Ridge, Illinois

Bud Fredericks, Ph.D.
Teaching Research,
Monmouth, Oregon

Jon F. Miller, Ph.D.
Communication Disorders
  Department,
Waisman Center on Mental
  Retardation and Human
  Development
University of Wisconsin,
Madison, Wisconsin

Carol Niman-Reed, M.S.,
  O.T.R.
Occupational Therapist
  Consultant,
St. Louis, Missouri

J. Dennis Odell, M.D.
Medical Director,
Developmental Center for
  Handicapped Persons,
Utah State University,
Logan, Utah

Siegfried M. Pueschel, M.D.,
Ph.D., M.P.H.
Director, Child Development
  Center,
Rhode Island Hospital;
Brown University—Program in
  Medicine,
Providence, Rhode Island

John E. Rynders, Ph.D.
Professor, Department of
  Educational Psychology,
Special Education Program,
University of Minnesota,
Minneapolis, Minnesota

Stuart J. Schleien,
Associate Professor,
Department of Physical Education
  and Therapeutic Recreation,
University of Minnesota,
Minneapolis, Minnesota

Dixie H. Sleight, M.A.T.,
O.T.R.
Outreach Coordinator,
St. John's Mercy Child
  Development Center,
St. Louis, Missouri

Carol Tingey, Ph.D.,
F.A.A.M.D.
Associate Professor,
Early Intervention Research
  Institute,
Utah State University,
Logan, Utah

Reed Warren, Ph.D.
Associate Professor, Biology
Developmental Center for
  Handicapped Persons,
Utah State University,
Logan, Utah

PART ONE

MEDICAL ISSUES

Down syndrome is not difficult to diagnose. The delivery room doctor is usually the first to recognize the physical characteristics of Down syndrome. Although most of these have no functional or behavioral significance, questions about appearance are often asked. Parents who have not seen other infants with Down syndrome usually do not see a resemblance between their child and other children who have Down syndrome. Parents and others are tempted to respond to statements about the shape of the baby's eyes or length of fingers as being unimportant to them or to their child. They are right, of course, mere appearance does not dictate behavior. However, physical symptoms are visual markers of the other conditions that can impact on development.

Infants, children and adults with Down syndrome share not only appearance, but physical conditions that need routine observation and sometimes treatment. Ongoing problems include dry skin, respiratory tract infections, and a tendency toward ear problems. Although Down syndrome is common enough that most physicians know something about it, it is rare enough that many physicians have never treated a patient with Down syndrome. Parents and other care providers, therefore, must be aware of the possible problems and ask that the physician examine the child for those conditions.

In this section the basic medical issues of Down syndrome are described. Chapter 1 summarizes the chromosome abnormalities and physical features present in children with Down syndrome. Information on medical treatments for some symptoms of Down syndrome is also included.

From here, the focus narrows to a specific health concern, that of immune system deficiency. Chapter 2 delves into the clinical findings that suggest individuals with Down syndrome may have defective immune systems, particularly evidenced by increased incidence of infection, a lifelong health concern.

Additional health problems related to Down syndrome are presented in Chapter 3, along with screening procedures used to detect their presence. Early identification of possible problems enables physicians and parents to make proper choices for ongoing healthcare programs to maximize the health potential of individuals with Down syndrome.

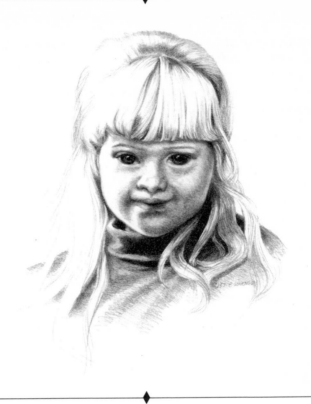

CHAPTER ONE

PHYSICAL CHARACTERISTICS, CHROMOSOME ANALYSIS, AND TREATMENT APPROACHES IN DOWN SYNDROME

SIEGFRIED M. PUESCHEL

♦

In this chapter, three main topics are discussed: the physical features of the child with Down syndrome; the chromosome aberrations observed in individuals with Down syndrome; and medical treatments that have been used to attempt to ameliorate the effects of Down syndrome.

PHYSICAL FEATURES OF THE CHILD WITH DOWN SYNDROME

Since John Langdon Down described the characteristics of the condition that bears his name, many articles have appeared in the literature reporting numerous features associated with this syndrome (Clark et al., 1978; Lee & Jackson, 1972; Singh, 1976; Strelling, 1976; Wahrman & Fried, 1970). More than 300 clinical signs have been described in children with Down syndrome (Coleman, 1978).

Since some of the characteristics occur with a high frequency, they are considered to be typical of this syndrome. It is important to recognize the clinical features in children with Down syndrome for diagnostic purposes; however, such physical characteristics are not identified on a regular basis in every child with Down syndrome, and none of the observed features can be considered to be specific for this chromosome disorder.

It is well known that the physical features of any human being are to a large extent determined by his or her genetic makeup. Therefore, children with Down syndrome will have some physical similarity to their parents since they receive their genes from both mother and father. Children with Down syndrome, however, will also have common features with other children who have the same chromosome disorder. The presence of three, instead of the normal two, 21 chromosomes is responsible for altered development during the early formation of the embryo and fetus. We do not know, however, in what way the additional chromosome material interferes with normal developmental sequences and how the structural changes are produced in the embryo. Moreover, we have no explanation of why some children with Down syndrome will display nearly all of the described features, whereas others will exhibit only a few of them.

Some characteristics, such as a single palmar crease and brachycephaly, can be observed at any age, whereas other physical features noted in persons with Down syndrome may change over time. For example, epicanthal folds or the initially abundant neck tissue will become less prominent as the child grows. On the other hand, such characteristics as the fissured tongue, skin changes, or dental anomalies, will become more apparent with increasing age.

Many of the physical features noted in children with Down syndrome are also observed at various frequencies in children with normal chromosomes. For example, 4–5 percent of children who do not have Down syndrome have a single palmar crease, 6–8 percent display epicanthal folds, and 26–43 percent exhibit overlapping of the helix of the ears (Holmes, 1976).

When physical features are discussed with parents, it should be stressed that many of the observed findings in Down syndrome do not cause any disability in the child. For example, the incurved little finger will not limit the function of the hand, nor will the slanting of the palpebral fissure interfere with the child's vision. Yet other defects, such as severe congenital heart disease or duodenal atresia, are serious and require prompt medical attention. It is also important to reassure parents that while physical changes will take place during the process of development and maturation, the features will not become worse over time. Parents should be made aware of the fact that children with Down syndrome are more similar to the average child in the community than they are different. The physician who is counseling parents should realize that the diagnosis of Down syndrome implies much more to the parents than the mere enumerations of various characteristics as it may exert a deep and far-reaching effect on each parent and the entire family. It is of utmost importance that the physician does not overemphasize the physical characteristics of the child,.but rather presents the infant with Down syndrome as a human being who needs nurturance and love.

In the subsequent discussion, some characteristics that can be identified on routine physical examination in children with Down syndrome are described.

Skull

The skull of the child with Down syndrome tends to be small, and the anterior-posterior diameter is shortened. According to Rett (1977), brachycephaly is found in 80% of children with Down syndrome. True microcephaly and hydrocephaly are rarely observed in Down syndrome. Benda (1969) reported that the head measurements in the newborn are within normal limits. However, Hall's studies (1964), as well as our investigations (Cronk, 1983), indicated that the mean head circumference of infants with Down syndrome is markedly below that of the age-equivalent child without Down syndrome but not in the microcephalic range.

In addition, children with Down syndrome reportedly have hypoplasia of their mid-facial bones. Strelling (1976) pointed to the size and grouping of the mid-facial features as a significant characteristic of the child with Down syndrome. He emphasized that the eyes, nose, and mouth are not only small, but are also grouped more closely together at the center of the face. In a quantitative study of the face, Fink, Madous, and Walker

(1975) found a significant degree of deficiency in mid-facial and mandibular areas in persons with Down syndrome. Lowe (1949) and Gerald and Silverman (1965) noted that the distance between the eyes is often reduced, the maxilla is underdeveloped, and the angle of the mandible may be somewhat obtuse. Benda (1969) reported abnormalities of the sphenoid bone, changes in the sella turcica, and displacement of the cribriform plate. Roche, Roche, and Lewis (1972) carried out a cephalometric x-ray study of the cranial base in 131 children and adults with Down syndrome and found a significant reduction in cranial base length. Another observation concerns the sinuses, which, according to Benda (1969), are underdeveloped.

Eyes

The eyes and features surrounding the eyes of the person with Down syndrome have attracted interest throughout the past century (Down, 1866; Brushfield, 1924; Lowe, 1949; Sequin 1866; Tredgold, 1908). Down (1866) observed that "the eyes are obliquely placed, and the internal canthi are more than normally distant from one another. The palpebral fissure is very narrow."

Prominent epicanthal folds are often noted in children with Down syndrome. These inner canthal skin folds may be prominent at the time of birth. However, as the child's nasal bridge develops, they become less apparent and sometimes may even disappear. Epicanthal folds have been reported to be present in 28–80 percent of individuals with Down syndrome (Gustavson, 1964; Hall, 1964; Lee & Jackson, 1972; Levinson, Friedman, & Stamps, 1955; Oster, 1953) in our study, 57 percent of the children had epicanthal folds (Pueschel, 1984).

The oblique placement of the palpebral fissures in Down syndrome is a common finding that was observed in 97 percent of young children with Down syndrome followed in a longitudinal study (Pueschel, 1984). Other investigators (Gustavson, 1964; Hall, 1964; Oster, 1953) have also noted the upward slant of the palpebral fissure to be a frequent sign in Down syndrome. In addition, the palpebral fissures are usually narrow (Benda, 1969).

Both hypertelorism and hypotelorism have been reported in persons with Down syndrome. The described variation in the distance between the eyes is primarily due to a lack of accurate measurements. Hypertelorism has been suggested because of the presence of a flat nasal bridge and marked epicanthal folds covering the inner canthi, making the distance between the eyes appear wide. Other observers have suggested the presence of a decreased distance between the inner canthi because of general hypoplasia of the mid-facial structures.

Hypotelorism in Down syndrome had already been observed in the beginning of the century by Barr (1904) and was later reported by

Brushfield (1924). Lowe (1949) reported that the distance between the inner canthi of persons with Down syndrome is approximately 1.5 cm less than in adults without Down syndrome.

Brushfield spots were noted by Down as fine white spots in the periphery of the iris. He brought this to the attention of Tredgold, who described this observation in 1908, long before Brushfield published his paper in 1924. Brushfield spots are white-gray protuberant areas on the surface of the iris. According to Purtscher (1958), these spots consist of connective tissue that is localized within the anterior layer of the iris. Benda (1969) thought that Brushfield spots were due to thinning of the iris stoma, as well as to abnormal pigment distribution.

In newborns with Down syndrome, Brushfield spots are not always identified. In one cohort of infants (Pueschel, 1984), Brushfield spots were observed in 75 percent. Other investigators reported the presence of Brushfield spots in Down syndrome to be between 30 and 70 percent (Gustavson, 1964; Hall, 1964; Lee & Jackson, 1972; Oster 1953). Singh (1976) found a higher percentage of Brushfield spots in white than in black persons with Down syndrome.

Nose

The nose of the child with Down syndrome is characterized by its reduced size and depression of the nasal bridge. The nares are sometimes anteverted, and the nostrils are narrow. Deviations of the nasal septum are common. The nasal bone is usually not ossified and is underdeveloped in the newborn. In one study (Pueschel, 1984), a hypoplastic nose was observed in 83% of newborn children with Down syndrome. Other investigators (Clark et al., 1978; Lee & Jackson, 1972; Wahrman & Fried, 1970) also described the flattening of the nasal bridge at a similar frequency, between 57.4 and 86.7 percent. The hypoplastic nose, in addition to the underdevelopment of the mid-facial region, makes the face of young children with Down syndrome appear flat. This flat facial profile has been emphasized as one of the most frequently observed characteristics (Hall, 1964).

Ears

An abnormal structure and reduction in the size of the ears are common findings in persons with Down syndrome. Thelander and Pryor (1966) and Aase, Wilson, and Smith (1973) reported shortened ears. Lower and oblique implantation of the ears occurring unilaterally or bilaterally have been described in young children with Down syndrome by Schmid (1976). In another study (Pueschel, 1984), an abnormal structure was observed in 28 percent of the children and low implantation of ears was found in 16 percent.

The most prominent finding is the overlapping or overfolding of the helix. This has been reported at a frequency between 28 and 78 percent (Clark et al., 1978; Domino & Newman, 1965; Gustavson 1964; Hall, 1964; Lee & Jackson, 1972; Levinson et al., 1955; Oster, 1953; Wahrman & Fried, 1970). It is of interest that this slightly broadened and downturned top of the helix has also been noted in many newborns without Down syndrome (Holmes, 1976). In addition to the overfolding of the helix, other structural ear anomalies include narrow ear canals, prominent antihelix, absent or attached earlobes, and projecting ears (Schmid, 1976).

Tongue

Some persons with Down syndrome keep the mouth open and the tongue protruding. Singh (1976) reported that protrusion of the tongue appears more often in white males (97 percent) than in white females (85 percent). He also reported a significant difference in the frequency of tongue protrusion when white males (92 percent) are compared with black males (67 percent).

In an attempt to explain tongue protrusion in persons with Down syndrome, it has been postulated that there is an absolute increase in the size of the tongue. Oster (1953) reported that 57 percent of children with Down syndrome had an enlarged tongue. Since it is difficult to measure the exact size of the tongue, Ardron, Harker, and Kemp (1972) assessed the size of the tongue roentgenographically. They did not observe a general enlargement of the tongue in children with Down syndrome, however, 5 of 8 children had some localized increase in tongue size near the lingual tonsil. Other investigators indicated that the underdeveloped maxilla, the narrow palate with broadened alveolar ridges, and the enlarged tonsils and adenoids render the oral cavity small (Barnes, 1923; Jenson, Cleal, & Yips, 1973).

Although Engler (1949) reported that all persons with Down syndrome over 5 years of age exhibit fissuring of the tongue, we have seen a number of older children who had normal-appearing tongues (Pueschel, 1984). The fissuring and papillary hypertrophy of the tongue are thought to be due to excessive sucking or chewing of the tongue.

Neck

The neck of the young child with Down syndrome appears to be short and broad. There is usually abundant skin and subcutaneous tissue in the posterior neck area of the newborn child. The base of the neck usually will stay broad, however, the increased tissue observed in the posterior neck will become less apparent as the child grows older.

Chest

The chest of the child with Down syndrome is usually normally shaped. The rib cage may appear somewhat shortened since in some children only 11 of the usual 12 ribs are present (Beber, 1965; Murray, Sylvester, & Gibson, 1966). An extensive study by Thuline and Islam (1966) found rib anomalies in 26 percent of females and 15 percent of males with Down syndrome. Some individuals had complete absence of the 12th rib, while others had a rudimentary 12th rib unilaterally or bilaterally.

Pectus excavatum was observed in 18 percent of children in our Down syndrome program and pectus carinatum was noted in 11 percent (Pueschel, 1984). Pectus excavatum was reported in 12 percent by Levinson et al. (1955) and in 6 percent by Domino and Newman (1965). Oster (1953) noted that both pectus excavatum and pectus carinatum were present in 5 percent of his study population. It is of note that these deformities of the sternum do not ordinarily interfere with respiratory or cardiovascular functions. Surgery is usually not indicated, since these are often only minor cosmetic defects.

Abdomen

In young children with Down syndrome, the abdomen often appears distended and enlarged, which is thought to be due to reduced muscle tone. In addition, diastasis recti is frequently observed. Levinson et al. (1955) reported diastasis recti in 76 percent of children with Down syndrome and Domino and Newman (1965) in 87 percent.

Umbilical hernias are not often reported in the literature. Levinson et al. (1955) and Domino and Newman (1965) observed a 4 percent and 6 percent frequency of umbilical hernias, respectively. A much higher prevalence of umbilical hernias was found in another study population; 89 percent of infants with Down syndrome had umbilical hernias measuring 2–25 mm in diameter (Pueschel, 1984). Benda (1969) recorded umbilical hernias in 90 percent of children, while Rett (1977) found umbilical hernias in 47 percent of his patients and inguinal hernias in 10 percent. This discrepancy among various observers is most likely due to the approach used in examining patients. If one merely describes the hernias noted on superficial visual inspection, one will not uncover the majority of hernias, which require careful palpation.

Extremities

The extremities of persons with Down syndrome are often described as short, particularly in their distal portions (Benda, 1969). Rett (1977) found that the metacarpal bones and the phalanges to be 10–30 percent shorter in children with Down syndrome than in children without Down syndrome. The hands and feet of children with Down syndrome have been described as broad and stubby.

Clinodactyly or brachyclinodactyly of the fifth finger is seen in approximately half of the individuals with Down syndrome (Benda, 1969). In one study (Pueschel, 1984), brachyclinodactyly of the left hand was observed in 51 percent of the children, whereas in the right hand it was noted in 50 percent. Similar findings were reported by Roche, Seward, and Sutherland (1961) and Oster (1953), who noted that 55 percent and 48 percent of children with Down syndrome respectively, had clinodactyly.

Brachyclinodactyly is thought to be due to a hypoplastic, slightly wedge-shaped, small middle phalanx of the fifth finger. Garn, Gall, and Nagy (1972) reported a hypoplastic middle phalanx in 21 percent of their study population, whereas Roche (1961) found this skeletal abnormality slightly more often (25 percent).

The single palmar transverse crease or the four-finger line at the mid-palmar surface of the hand has attracted special attention as a diagnostic sign in Down syndrome. It should be noted, however, that a single palmar crease is not present in every child with Down syndrome. Reports from the literature indicate that 42–64 percent of children with Down syndrome have a single transverse palmar crease (Clark et al., 1978; Domino & Newman, 1965; Gustavson, 1964; Hall, 1964; Lee & Jackson, 1972; Levinson et al., 1955; Oster, 1953; Wahrman & Fried, 1970).

Partial or complete syndactyly has also been reported at a higher frequency in children with Down syndrome than in those without. In one study (Pueschel, 1984), 10.7 percent of children displayed partial or complete syndactyly at both hands and feet. Hanhart (1960) noted syndactyly between toes in 2.1 percent, and Beckman, Gustavson, and Akesson (1962) observed syndactyly in 11.4 percent.

Dignan (1973) reported infrequent occurrence of polydactyly in Down syndrome. Three patients with partial adactyly, where the second, third, and fourth digits were absent from one hand only were seen by Pueschel and O'Donnell (1974). Since their report on unilateral partial adactyly in Down syndrome were published, four more patients with this hand malformation have been encountered.

A wide space between first and second toes is a frequent observation and was recorded in 96 percent of Pueschel's patients (1984). In addition, a plantar (sole of foot) crease is often found between the first and second toes (94 percent).

Summary

Although there are many other signs and symptoms that characterize the person with Down syndrome, the most important external phenotypic features have been discussed above. It should be emphasized again that the phenotypic expression in Down syndrome is of primary significance for the physician in establishing the clinical diagnosis. The observed features, however, are usually not a functional handicap and do not render the children unattractive. It is of importance to recognize that beyond the characteristics there is first and foremost a child who is endowed with significance and worth.

CHROMOSOME ANALYSIS

In the 1930s, some physicians suspected that chromosome problems might be the cause of Down syndrome (Fanconi, 1939; Waardenburg, 1932). At that time, however, the technology for examining chromosomes was not advanced enough to test this theory. Only in the mid 1950s did methods to study chromosomes become available (Tjio & Levan, 1956). This led to the discovery by Lejeune, Gauthier, and Turpin (1959) that children with Down syndrome had one extra small chromosome. These French investigators noted 47 chromosomes in each cell instead of the normal 46 chromosomes; instead of the usually observed two 21 chromosomes, they found three 21 chromosomes. As Fig. 1-1 shows, the chromosomes are arranged in pairs. However, as indicated by the arrow, in the 21 group there are three chromosomes. Approximately 95 percent of children with Down syndrome have this chromosome makeup, trisomy 21.

There are two other chromosome problems observed in children with Down syndrome. In approximately 4–5 percent of children, the extra 21 chromosome is attached to another chromosome, usually a chromosome 14, 21, or 22, which is referred to as translocation. In this situation, the total count of chromosomes will be 46 because two chromosomes are attached to each other, as indicated in Fig. 1-2. Again, the total number of chromosomes 21 is three, which, as we know, will bring about the features of Down syndrome.

It is important to find out whether or not a child with translocation Down syndrome has a parent who is a carrier. If one of the parents is a carrier, there is an increased risk that this parent will have more children with Down syndrome and needs genetic counseling.

The third type of chromosome problem, which is least commonly observed in children with Down syndrome, is called *mosaicism*. It occurs in approximately 1 percent of children with Down syndrome. Mosaicism

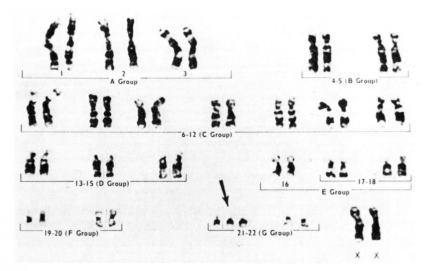

Figure 1-1. Shown are the chromosomes (karyotype) of a girl with Down syndrome. Note the extra 21 chromosome (arrow).

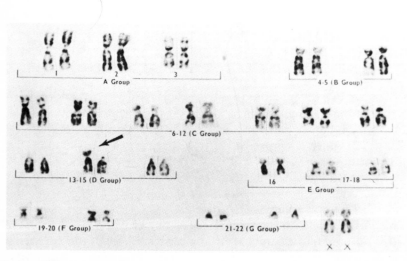

Figure 1-2. Shown is a karyotype of a girl with translocation Down syndrome. The arrow indicates the extra 21 chromosome, which is translocated or attached to a 14 chromosome.

is thought to be due to an error in one of the first cell divisions shortly after conception, as noted in Fig. 1–3. When the baby is born, there are usually some cells with 47 chromosomes and other cells with the normal 46 chromosomes, presenting a kind of "mosaic picture."

Regardless whether it is trisomy 21, translocation, or mosaicism, it is always the presence of three 21 chromosomes that is responsible for the specific physical features and the mental deficiencies observed in the majority of children with Down syndrome.

During the past decades, new methods in visualizing details of individual chromosomes have allowed the identification of children who only have parts of additional chromosome 21 material. Using these new banding techniques, it was found that it is not the entire extra chromosome 21 but only a small segment of its long arm that causes Down syndrome. It is not known, however, in what way this extra chromosome material interferes with the development of the embryo and fetus or how the extra genes result in abnormal brain function.

During the past century, many investigators have speculated about the cause of Down syndrome. Although it is not known why chromosomes

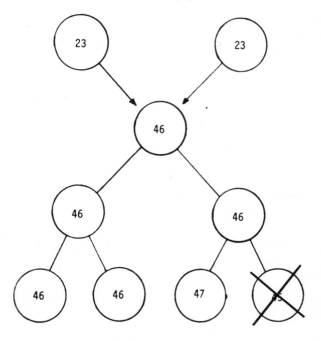

Figure 1–3. In mosaicism, the nondisjunction is thought to occur during one of the early cell divisions. When this infant is born, there will be some cells with 46 chromosomes and others with 47 chromosomes. Cells with 45 or fewer chromosomes usually do not survive.

do not divide properly (Fig. 1-4), new theories of causation have been developed in recent years. It has been postulated that exposure to x-rays, viral infections, or certain potent drugs and/or hormonal and immunological problems may be responsible for the chromosome anomaly in Down syndrome (Crowley, Hayden, & Gulati 1983).

Previously, mothers were often blamed for bringing children with Down syndrome into the world since it is well known that there is a relationship between maternal age and incidence of Down syndrome, i.e., the older the mother, the greater the risk of giving birth to a child with Down syndrome. Recent reports, however, indicate that there may also be a relationship between the father's age and the incidence of Down syndrome; however, this relationship is less well established (Hook, 1983). In studies done during the past decade examining chromosomes from both parents, it was found that in at least 20–30 percent of cases, the extra chromosome 21 comes from the father (Thuline & Pueschel, 1983).

THERAPEUTIC APPROACHES FOR CHILDREN WITH DOWN SYNDROME

In order to improve physical features and mental functioning in children with Down. syndrome, a multitude of medical treatment modalities, including hormones, vitamins, sicca cells, minerals, and various combinations thereof, have been introduced during the past decades.

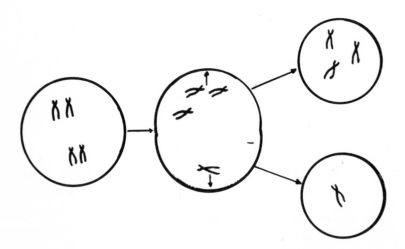

Figure 1–4. During the process of cell division, two 21 chromosomes "stick together" (nondisjunction). In the following cell generation, one cell will have one chromosome less (this is not a variable cell) and the other cell will have one additional chromosome. (For demonstration purposes, only two pairs of chromosomes are shown here.)

Thyroid Hormone

It is assumed that the first reported treatment was carried out at the end of the last century when T. T. Smith (1896) administered thyroid hormone extract to children with Down syndrome. Since then, many physicians have provided thyroid hormone to persons with Down syndrome and other retardation syndromes. Koch, Share, and Graliker (1965), who studied the effect of thyroid therapy in children with Down syndrome, did not find any significant difference in the overall functioning of the groups of Down syndrome children receiving thyroid hormone, placebo, and no treatment.

Pituitary Extract

Pituitary extract has been employed in the treatment of children with Down syndrome. While claims have been made of marked improvement in treated children, Berg, Kirman, Stern, and Mittwoch (1961), as well as Diamond and Moon (1961), reported that pituitary extract given to children with Down syndrome did not benefit their intellectual and social development.

Glutamic Acid

Glutamic acid and its derivatives have been used in the treatment of children with Down syndrome and other developmental disabilities since the 1940s. Many workers found this compound to be beneficial to children with Down syndrome, yet investigations by Lombard, Gilbert, and Donofrio (1955) and as Astin and Ross (1960) reported no significant improvement after glutamic acid administration to children with Down syndrome and other developmental disabilities.

Dimethylsulfoxide

Dimethylsulfoxide also has been advocated in the treatment of children with mental retardation. In particular, Chilean investigators have claimed marked improvement in the overall functioning of children with Down syndrome following the administration of dimethylsulfoxide (Aspillage, Morizon, & Avendano, 1975). However, the many methodologic inadequacies of this study render the results uninterpretable. In 1973, a short-term study was carried out in Oregon to assess the effects of dimethylsulfoxide on behavior and academic achievement in retarded individuals, including children with Down syndrome. This study revealed that there was no significant improvement of the observed variables in the children after administration of dimethylsulfoxide (Gabourie, Becker, & Bateman, 1975).

Sicca Cells

In the 1930s, sicca cell therapy was introduced and is still used since in certain parts of Europe. This form of treatment consists of injecting lyophilized material prepared from embryonic animal organs. It has been hypothesized that this will stimulate the growth and function of the corresponding tissues in the human body (Schmid, 1976). Black, Kato, and Walker (1966) conducted a double-blind study in order to evaluate the effects of sicca cell therapy. These investigators found no evidence that such treatment was of any value to the children's overall development. Another study, conducted by Bardon (1964), also did not find a significant difference between the experimental and control groups; thus, Bardon concluded that sicca cell therapy is completely ineffective in the treatment of children with Down syndrome.

5-Hydroxytryptophan

Since Tu and Zellweger (1965) reported low blood serotonin concentrations in children with Down syndrome, several investigators have employed the precursor of serotonin, 5-hydroxytryptophan, in the treatment of children with Down syndrome. Bazelon et al. (1967) observed improvement in muscle tone, tongue protrusion, and activity level in infants with Down syndrome who had been given 5-hydroxytryptophan. In a follow-up study using a double-blind design and comparing children with Down syndrome who received 5-hydroxytryptophan with a placebo group, no significant difference in the developmental parameters of children in the two groups was found. Also, Partington, MacDonald, and Tu (1971) and Weise, Koch, Shaw, and Rosenfeld (1974), who gave 5-hydroxytryptophan to children with Down syndrome, did not observe behavioral differences between treated and nontreated children. Pueschel (1984) undertook a comprehensive study of young children with Down syndrome, evaluating the effect of 5-hydroxytryptophan administration on motor, intellectual, social, and language developments and did not uncover a significant beneficial effect using 5-hydroxytryptophan and/or vitamin B_6.

Vitamins

Vitamin treatment, in particular treatment with vitamin E and vitamin B_6, has been provided to children with Down syndrome. Coleman (1973), who studied the effect of vitamin B_6 administration, did not observe a significant improvement in intellectual functioning of the treated children. The only beneficial results related to fewer infections and improved growth rate of children receiving vitamin B_6.

There have been numerous therapeutic approaches with various combinations of vitamins in addition to hormones, enzymes, minerals, and other substances. In Germany, Haubold (1967) recommended a mixture of vitamins, hormones, and minerals, which he called *basis therapy*. White and Kaplitz (1964), who treated children with Down syndrome according to Haubold's instructions, did not find any significant improvement of the treated children, however.

In this country, Turkel (1975) has treated hundreds of children with the *U-series*, which is comprised of nearly 50 different compounds, including hormones, vitamins, minerals, enzymes, and others. Turkel claimed that the child's physical features as well as intellectual functioning can be improved by administering the U-series. Bumbalo, Morelewicz, and Berens (1964) investigated the effects of the U-series in children with Down syndrome in a double-blind study. No beneficial effects were observed in children in the treatment group.

An article in the *Proceedings of the National Academy of Science*, with the title "Can nutritional supplements help mentally retarded children?," has brought the subject of multiple-vitamin treatment in large doses into the limelight (Harrell, Capp, Davis, Peerless, & Ravitz, 1981). Results of this study have been widely publicized in the lay press. The authors reported that five of six children who received a nutritional supplement that included 8 minerals and 11 vitamins increased their average IQ score by 5.0–9.6 points, whereas the 11 subjects who had been given a placebo showed negligible changes during the 4-month study. During the second 4-month period, the subjects who had been given a placebo received the nutritional supplements, and their IQ score increased an average of 10.2 points. The investigators reported that three of four children with Down syndrome had gains of 10–25 IQ points. These children allegedly also showed physical changes toward normal.

A thorough review of this article, however, found that the overall study design was rather poor: there was not random assignment to study and control groups; there was an unequal distribution of children in the study and control groups; no mention was made of whether the vitamin-mineral supplement was indistinguishable from the placebo in taste, smell, and visual appearance; compliance was not objectively tested; the study was not controlled for seizures, unusual behaviors, vision, and hearing impairments; and unconventional methods were used for testing the thyroid function of the children in the study.

Several subsequent investigations have failed to reproduce the results of Harrell et al. Weathers (1983) treated 24 children with Down syndrome, ages 6–17, for 4 months with the same dose of minerals and vitamins as used by Harrell's group (1981). A matched control group of 23 children received a placebo. Measures of IQ, visual-motor integration, height, weight, and behavior ratings by parents failed to show significant differences between the two groups. Since Harrell et al. had reported that most of the improvements were noted in the younger subjects, Weathers divided his subjects into age groupings of 6–8, 9–12, 13–17 years; however, there were still no significant differences among the age groups. Bennett, McClelland, Kriegsman, Brazee, and Sells (1983) also evaluated the treatment effect using Harrell's vitamin-mineral mixture in a double-blind case-control study involving 20 home-reared children with Down syndrome between 5 and 13 years old. Following an 8-month study, these investigators did not uncover a significant difference between the treatment and placebo groups in IQ, school achievement, speech and language function, and neuromotor competence. Smith, Spiker, Peterson, Cicchetti, and Justine (1984) reported a similar study. These investigators did not find any notable gains in measured intellectual functioning of school-aged children with Down syndrome who received the vitamin-mineral formula for an 8-month period.

Summary

Although no effective medical treatments are available at the present time, people with Down syndrome should be afforded appropriate medical services (see Chapter 3), and specialized educational services (see Chapters 7–12). Furthermore, their appearance, attire, and general hygiene should be such as to enhance their acceptance and integration into society. People with Down syndrome must be accepted and offered a status that acknowledges their rights, privileges, and responsibilities as family members and as citizens.

REFERENCES

Aase, J.M., Wilson, A.C., & Smith, D.W. (1973). Small ears in Down syndrome: A helpful diagnostic aid. *Journal of Pediatrics, 82,* 845.

Andron, G.M., Harker, P., & Kemp, F.H. (1972). Tongue size in Down syndrome. *Journal of Mental Deficiency, 16,* 160–166.

Aspillage, M.J., Morizon, G., Avendano, I. (1975). Dimethyl sulfoxide therapy in severe retardation in mongoloid children. *Ann. NY: Acad. Sci, 243,* 421–431.

Astin, A.W., Ross, S. (1960). Glutamic acid and human intelligence. *Psychology Bulletin, 57,* 429–434.

Bardon, L. M. (1964). Sicca cell treatment in mongolism. *Lancet, 2,* 234–235.

Barnes, N.P. (1923). Mongolism: Importance of early recognition and treatment. *Ann. Clin. Med., 1,* 302.

Barr, M.W. (1904). Mental defectives: Their history, treatment, and training. London: Rebman.

Bazelon, M., Paine, R.S., Cowie, V.A., Hunt, P. et al. (1967). Reversal of hypotonia in infants with Down's syndrome by administration of 5-hydroxytryptophan. *Lancet, 1,* 1130.

Beber, B.A. (1965). Absence of a rib in Down syndrome. *Lancet, 2,* 289.

Beckman, L., Gustavson, K.H., & Akesson, H.O. (1962). Studies of some morphological traits in mental defectives. *Hereditas, 48,* 105.

Benda, C.E. (1969). *Down syndrome: Mongolism and its management.* New York: Grune & Stratton.

Bennett, F.C., McClelland, S., Kriegsmann, F.A., Brazee, A., & Sells, C.J. (1983). Vitamin and mineral supplementation in Down syndrome. *Pediatrics, 72,* 707-713.

Berg, J.M., Kirman, B.H., Stern, J., & Mittwoch, U. (1961). Treatment of mongolism. *Journal of Mental Science, 107,* 475-480.

Black, D.B., Kato, J.G., & Walker, G.W.H. (1966). A study of improvement in mentally retarded children accruing from sicca cell therapy. *American Journal of Mental Deficiency, 70,* 499-508.

Brushfield, T. (1924). Mongolism. *British Journal of Child Disorders, 21,* 241.

Bumbalo, T.S., Morelewicz, H.V., & Berens, D.L. (1964). Treatment of Down's syndrome with the "U" series of drugs. *JAMA, 5,* 187.

Down, J.L. (1866). Observations on an ethnic classification of idiots. *London Hospital Clinic Lecture Reports, 3,* 259-262.

Clark, R.M. (1929). The mongol: A new explanation. *Journal of Mental Science, 75,* 261.

Coleman, M. (1978). Down's syndrome. *Pediatric Annals, 7* 90-103.

Cronk, C.E. (1983). Anthropometric studies. In S.M. Pueschel (Ed), *A study of the young child with Down syndrome.* New York: Human Science Press.

Crowley, P.H., Hayden, T.L. & Gulati, D.K. (1983). Etiology of Down syndrome. In S.M. Pueschel & J.E. Rynders (Eds), *Down syndrome: Advances in biomedicine and the behavioral sciences.* Cambridge, MA: Ware Press.

Diamond, E.F. & Moon, M.S. (1961). Neuromuscular development in mongoloid children. *American Journal of Mental Deficiency, 66,* 218.

Dignan, P. St. J. (1973). Polydactyly in Down's syndrome. *American Journal of Mental Deficiency, 77,* 486.

Domino, G. & Newman, D. (1965). Relationships of physical stigmata to intellectual subnormality in mongoloids. *American Journal of Mental Deficiency, 69,* 541.

Engler, M. (1949). *Mongolism (peristaltic amenia).* London: Wright.

Fanconi, G. (1939). Die Mutationstheorie des Mongolismus. *Schweizerische Medizinische Wochenschrift, 69,* 81-83.

Fink, G.B., Madous, W.K., & Walker, G.F. (1975). A quantitative study of the face in Down syndrome. *American Journal Orthodontics, 69,* 540-553.

Gabourie, J., Becker, J.W., & Bateman, B. (1975). Oral dimethyl sulfoxide in mental retardation. Part I: Preliminary behavioral and psychometric data. Annals of the New York Academy of Science, *243,* 1-508.

Garn, S.M., Gall, J.C. Jr., & Nagy, J.M. (1972). Brachymesophalangia-5 without cone-epiphysis mid-5 in Down's syndrome. *American Journal of Physical Anthropology, 36,* 253-255.

Gerald, B.E., & Silverman, F.C. (1965). Normal and abnormal interorbital distances with special reference to mongolism. *American Journal of Roentgenology, 95,* 154-161.

Gustavson, K.H. (1964). *Down's syndrome: A clinical and cytogenetic investigation.* Uppsala, Sweden: Almqvist & Wiksell.

Hall, B. (1964). *Mongolism in newborns—A clinical and cytogenetic study.* Lund: Berlingska Boktryckeriet.

Hanhart, E. (1960). 800 Falle von Mongoloidismus in konstitutioneller Betrachtung. Arch. Julius Klaus-Stift. *Vererbungsforschung, Sozialanthropologie & Rassenhygiene, 35*, 1.

Harrell, R.F., Capp, R.H., Davis, D.R., Peerless, J., & Ravitz, L.R. (1981). Can nutritional supplements help mentally retarded children? An exploratory study. *Proceedings of the National Academy of Science, 78*, 574–578.

Haubold, H. (1967). Beeinflussung des phenotyps mongoloider Kinder durch ein fruheinsetzende Dauerbehandlung. *Anesthetische Meduzin, 13*, 3.

Holmes, L.B. (1976). *The malformed newborn: Practical perspectives.* Boston: Developmental Disabilities Council.

Hook, E.B. (1983). Epidemiology of Down syndrome. In S.M. Pueschel & J.E. Rynders (Eds.), *Down syndrome: Advances in biomedicine and the behavioral sciences.* Cambridge, MA: Ware Press.

Jensen, G.M., Cleal, J.F., & Yips, A.S.G. (1973). Dentoalvealor morphology and developmental changes in Down syndrome (trisomy 21). *American Journal of Orthodontics, 64*, 607.

Koch, R., Share, J., & Graliker, B. (1965). The effects of cytomel on young children with Down's syndrome (mongolism): A double-blind longitudinal study. *Journal of Pediatrics, 66*, 776.

Lee, L., & Jackson, J. (1972). Diagnosis of Down's syndrome: Clinical vs. laboratory. *Clinical Pediatrics, 11*, 353–356.

Lejeune, J., Gauthier, M., & Turpin, R. (1959). Les chromosomes humains en culture de tissus. *Comptes Rendus de L Academie des Sciences (Paris)*, 248–602.

Levinson, A., Friedman, A., & Stamps, F. (1955). Variability of mongolism. *Pediatrics, 16*, 43.

Lombard, J.P., Gilbert, J.G., & Donofrio, A.F. (1955). The effects of glutamic acid upon the intelligence, social maturity, and adjustment of a group of mentally retarded children. *American Journal of Mental Deficiency, 60*, 122–132.

Lowe, R. (1949). Eyes in mongolism. *British Journal of Ophthalmology, 33*, 131–174.

Murray, J.B., Sylvester, P.E., & Gibson, J. (1966). Rib absence in Down's syndrome. *Lancet, 1*, 1375.

Oster, J. (1953). *Mongolism: A clinico-geneological investigation comprising 526 mongols living in Seeland and neighboring islands of Denmark.* Copenhagen: Danish Science Press.

Partington, M.W., MacDonald, M.R.A., & Tu, J.B. (1971). 5-Hydroxytryptophan (5-HTP) in Down's syndrome. *Developmental Medicine and Child Neurology, 13*, 362–372.

Pueschel, S.M. (1984). *The young child with Down syndrome.* New York: Human Science Press.

Pueschel, S.M., & O'Donnell, P. (1974). Unilateral partial adactyly in Down's syndrome. *Pediatrics, 54*, 466–469.

Purtscher, E. (1958). Knotenformige Verdichtungen im Irisstroma bei Mongolismus. *Von Graefes Archive der Ophthalmologic, 160*, 200.

Rett, A. (1977). *Mongolismus*. Bern: Huber.

Roche, A.F. (1961). Clinodactyly and brachymesophalangia of the fifth finger. *Acta Paediatrics, 50,* 387.

Roche, A.F., Roche, R.J., & Lewis, A.B. (1972). The cranial base in trisomy 21. *Journal of Mental Deficiency Research, 16,* 7–20.

Roche, A.F., Seward, F.S., & Sutherland, S. (1961). Nonmetrical observations on cranial roentgenograms in mongolism. *American Journal of Roentgenology, 84,* 659–662.

Schmid, F. (1976). *Das Mongolismus-Syndrom*. Muensterdorf: Hansen and Hansen.

Sequin, E. (1866). *Idiocy and its treatment by the physiological method*. New York: Wood.

Singh, D.M. (1976). Down's syndrome: A study of clinical features. *Journal of the National Medical Association, 68,* 521–524.

Smith, G.F., Spiker, D., Peterson, C.P., Cicchetti, D., & Justine, P. (1984). Use of megadoses of vitamins with minerals in Down syndrome. *Journal of Pediatrics, 105,* 228–234.

Smith, T.T. (1896). A peculiarity in the shape of the hand in idiots of the mongol type. *Pediatrics, 2,* 315–320.

Strelling, M.K. (1976). Diagnosis of Down's syndrome at birth. *British Medical Journal, 2,* 1386.

Thelander, H.E., & Pryor, H.B. (1966). Abnormal patterns of growth and development in mongolism: An anthropometric study. *Clinical Pediatrics, 5,* 493.

Thuline, H.C., & Islam, A.R. (1966). Absence of a rib in Down's syndrome. *Lancet, 1,* 1156.

Thuline, H.C., & Pueschel, S.M. (1983). Cytogentics in Down syndrome. In S.M. Pueschel & J.E. Rynders (Eds.), *Down syndrome: Advances in biomedicine and the behavioral sciences*. Cambridge, MA: Ware Press.

Tjio, J.H., & Levan, A. (1956). The chromosome number of man. *Hereditas, 42,* 1–6.

Tredgold, R.F. (1908). *Mental deficiency (amentia)*. London: Bailliere, Tindall, & Cox.

Tu, J., & Zellweger, J. (1965). Blood serotonin deficiency in Down's syndrome. *Lancet, 2,* 715.

Turkel, H. (1975). Medical amelioration of Down's syndrome incorporating the orthomolecular approach. *Journal of Ortho-Molec Psychiatry, 4,* 102–115.

Waardenburg, P.J. (1932). *Das menschliche Auge und seine Erbanlagen*. The Hague: Nijhoff.

Wahrman, J. (1970). The Jerusalem prospective newborn survey of mongols. *Annals of the New York Academy of Science, 171,* 341–360.

Weathers, C. (1983). Effects of nutritional supplementation on IQ and certain other variables associated with Down syndrome. *American Journal of Mental Deficiency, 88,* 214–217.

Weise, P., Koch, R., Shaw, K.N.F., & Rosenfeld, M.J. (1974). The use of 5-HTP in the treatment of Down's syndrome. *Pediatrics, 54,* 165.

White, D., & Kaplitz, S.W. (1964). Treatment of Down's syndrome with a vitamin mineral hormone preparation. *Int. Copenhagen Cong. Sci. Study Ment. Retard, 1,* 224.

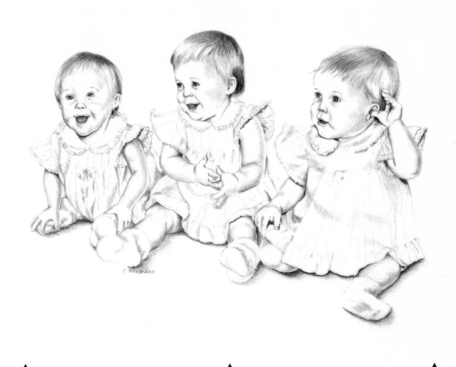

CHAPTER TWO

IMMUNE DEFICIENCY IN DOWN SYNDROME

REED WARREN

A number of clinical findings suggest an abnormal or defective immune system in Down syndrome. Patients with Down syndrome have an increased incidence of infections, with infections of the respiratory tract (lungs, bronchi, etc.) being more than 100 times more frequent in children with Down syndrome than in age-matched control children (Levin et al, 1979). The death rate from respiratory infections in Down syndrome is particularly high during the first year of life and remains significantly elevated through the age of 5 (Deaton, 1973). Also, mothers of patients with Down syndrome have an increased frequency of antibodies against thyroid tissue (Burgio, Severi, Rossoni, & Vaccaro, 1965). In order to understand what this means, it is necessary to understand the immune system.

THE IMMUNE SYSTEM

The immune system is of vital importance to the body. This system is made up of several kinds of specialized white blood cells which recognize and eliminate foreign substances such as bacteria and viruses. The various white blood cells of the immune system are manufactured in bone marrow, but they move out to live and work in other parts of the body.

Most people do not suffer twice from diseases such as measles, chicken pox, or mumps, because a first encounter with the organisms that cause these diseases triggers a response in the body that enables a second response to be faster and more robust.

The immune response to a bout of German measles protects the body from measles viruses encountered later in life, the body remembers that it has previously encountered the virus, and the body is protected from that virus but not from others.

White Blood Cells

Lymphocytes are white blood cells that are an essential component in all immune responses. Lymphocytes travel from the bloodstream, through the tissues, and back into the blood. These cells may be divided into two major groups: T lymphocytes (T cells) and B lymphocytes (B cells).

T cells are responsible for T cell–type immunity. They are named after the thymus, a gland at the base of the neck. The thymus is a grayish organ with two lobes located high in the thoracic cavity just above the heart. The thymus is a special place where T cells mature so that they can function in the immune response. Immature T cells are formed by cell division in the bone marrow; the cells then travel to the thymus where they undergo changes that allow them to play their normal role in the immune system. If the thymus is removed from a young mammal shortly after birth, the animal will grow up with a very reduced immune capability. B cells are produced by cell division in the bone marrow. The cells remain in the marrow for some time where they mature and become ready to perform their important function of producing antibodies.

T Cell (Cellular Immune System)

Many of the reactions and processes of the immune response take place in lymphoid tissue located in the small lymph nodes in the body and in the spleen. T cells recognize and destroy foreign cells or any of the body's own cells that have been altered by virus infections, cancer, or old age. The T cell has a special structure (receptor) on its cell surface that recognizes and reacts to foreign cells or altered cells of the body. The type of T cell that actually attacks foreign and altered cells is the cytotoxic T cell (or the killer T cell). Killer T cells make it difficult to perform certain types of organ or tissue transplantation because these cells recognize and mobilize an attack on the foreign material.

B Cell (Humoral Immune Responses)

Humoral immunity, the body's other main immune defense against pathogenic bacteria and viruses, depends on B cells. In response to a bacteria or virus (antigen), some B cells will manufacture antibodies. Each antibody has a specific ability to combine with a specific antigen. Combining of antibodies with antigen result in the elimination of the antigen from the body. When antibodies are mixed with antigens in a test tube, the antibodies attach to the antigen's three-dimensional shape in a way similar to a key fitting in a lock.

The closer the fit between the molecular shapes of the two molecules, the stronger the binding between them and the greater the strength of the antibody with that antigen. Specificity is not absolute, and some antibodies can bind with many different antigens. The human body contains antibodies to as many as one million different antigens.

If an antigen is injected into an experimental animal for the first time, at least one of the thousands of different types of antibodies in the blood can bind to this antigen to some extent. The antigen is then ingested onto a larger cell (macrophage). The larger cell travels through the body, including the lymph nodes, where hundreds of B cells reside. Each B cell bears on its surface a sample of the antibody it synthesizes, and the bacterial antigen on the large cell's surface will bind to the B cells with a corresponding antibody. The binding of an antigenic macrophage stimulates a lymphocyte to divide, forming identical new cells, all of which produce identical antibodies. Helper T cells are vital to antibody synthesis and new cell formation. Some new B cells travel to other lymph nodes and begin to produce antibodies. Within a few days of the initial infection, a great amount of the antibody appears in the blood.

ACTIVELY ACQUIRED IMMUNITY

The large amount of antibody secreted into the bloodstream at the time of the body's first exposure to a bacterial antigen is the primary immune response to the antigen. Following the primary response, the antigen will eventually disappear from the blood, bound by antibody and engulfed by larger cells that ingest the antigen. Suppressor T cells then cause the cells that are producing antibodies to stop dividing. However, the new cells do not die out; rather, they remain in the body as an enlarged population of cells that can react to that particular antigen. If the same bacterial antigen enters the body again, a secondary immune response, faster and more extensive than the primary response, occurs to repel the antigen.

The identical cells of lymphocytes formed during the primary response to an antigen constitute the body's memory of that antigen. Because each lymphocyte produces only one type (or, at most, a few types) of antibody, the body must build up an identical copy for each antigen it encounters before it has an arsenal against most of the microorganisms it encounters. Babies have many colds and infections in their first few years because they must encounter many new antigens and build up many memory cells before they can become immune to as many diseases as the average adult.

A primary response can come from illness or from microorganisms from another source being injected into the body, as in vaccination. A primary immune response creates identical cells ready to trigger a secondary response at the next appearance of the disease antigen. Medical researchers have developed vaccines for a number of bacterial and viral diseases, including polio and influenza. "Booster shots" serve to jog the body's immunological memory into producing more antibodies and more cells, ensuring that there are plenty of memory cells available if a pathogen should invade.

PASSIVELY ACQUIRED IMMUNITY

People are passively immune when they contain antibodies that were not produced in their own bodies. For example, newborn babies are passively immune, temporarily protected from disease by antibodies that reached them from their mothers' blood before birth. These maternal antibodies are steadily used up over a period of a few months until the babies' immune systems are sufficiently mature to take over.

Breast-fed infants are also protected by colostrum, a thin fluid produced by the mammary glands after childbirth before the flow of milk begins. Colostrum contains antibodies believed to protect the human infant's digestive tract from infections. Human babies do not absorb antibodies from colostrum into the blood, although the young of some other mammals do.

AUTOIMMUNITY

Autoimmunity is a condition in which the immune system reacts against its own antigens. Normally, the immune system learns to distinguish "self" from "nonself" during development, and thus it does not respond to itself. Occasionally, however, the self recognition system breaks down. Usually we do not know why this happens. An example of an autoimmune disease is rheumatic fever, in which autoimmune reactions break down the body's proteins, particularly in the heart. Antibodies that react with self tissue are termed autoantibodies. Rheumatoid arthritis and a number of other devastating, although fairly rare, diseases are also thought to be caused by autoantibodies.

IMMUNE DEFICIENCY IN DOWN SYNDROME

Childhood Leukemia

The incidence of lymphocytic (childhood) leukemia is about 18 times higher in children with Down syndrome than it is in children without this syndrome (Burgio et al., 1965; Scoll, Stein, & Hansen, 1982). This finding provides additional strong evidence for immune system abnormalities in Down syndrome. Leukemia is a form of cancer that involves the leukocytes or white blood cells. Leukemic cells differ from normal cells in two main ways: they divide more rapidly, and they dedifferentiate, that is, they look as if they have reverted to an early stage in their development.

As leukemic cells divide and dedifferentiate, changes occur in their membranes resulting in recognizable nonself antigenic structures than can be recognized by the cellular immune system. Many immunologists believe that cancer cells, including leukemic cells, appear rather often in the body but are usually eliminated by the immune system. It is possible that the cellular immune system developed principally as a weapon, an immune surveillance system, against cancers. Therefore, that children with Down syndrome have an increased incidence of leukemia is evidence for a defect in their cellular immune system.

Deficiency in the Thymus

In 1965, Benda and Strassman noted abnormalities of the thymus in Down syndrome. This was before the role of the thymus in the immune system was understood. As described earlier, the thymus is the place in the body where T cells go to develop into mature cells able to participate in the immune response. We now know that many patients with Down syndrome have small and abnormal thymuses, with contracted and depleted cortexes (the specific tissue where T cells mature) (Levin et al., 1979). These deficiencies are especially prominent in newborn infants with Down syndrome who die shortly after birth; the deficiencies become less marked in thymuses of older patients with Down syndrome.

It is not surprising that thymus deficiencies are more pronounced in young patients with Down syndrome. Most of the functions of the normal thymus are carried out early in a person's life, and the thymus becomes less important as the person becomes older—as long as the other parts of the immune system remain functional. In fact, after about the time of puberty, the thymus begins to shrink and, as time goes by, becomes tiny and nonfunctional.

T Cell-Mediated Immunity in Down Syndrome

Studies show that people with Down syndrome, including newborns and young children, have reduced numbers of T cells—usually not more than 60 percent of normal (Levin et al., 1979). Strong evidence also exists that these T cells do not function normally (Levin et al., 1979; Whittingham, Pitt, Shauna, & MacKay, 1977). Several studies have found that people with Down syndrome also have deficiencies in their responses to antigens injected into the skin (Szigeti, R., Revesz, & Schuler, 1974).

It has been suggested that deficient responses of T cells in patients with Down syndrome may be caused by excessive activity of suppressor T cells, preventing other T cells from responding, or by reduced helper T cell function (Levin et al., 1979; Noble & Warren, 1987a, 1987b).

Humoral Immunity in Down Syndrome

Despite definite deficiency of T cell–mediated immunity in Down syndrome, humoral or B cell–mediated immunity appears, in general, to be quite normal. Some researchers have reported minor differences in the levels of antibodies (Levin et al., 1979), but these differences do not appear to be clinically relevant and do not correlate with an increased incidence of infections in Down syndrome. Also, it is difficult to know if these minor differences reflect actual defects in B cell immunity, per se, or if they are an indirect indication of a deficiency in T cell "help." A lack of T cell help could result in abnormalities in antibody production despite normal B cell numbers and function.

Natural Killer Cell Function in Down Syndrome

The natural killer cell is a type of lymphocyte that is neither a T cell nor a B cell. It is called the natural killer cell because it kills malignant or virally transformed target cells without prior exposure to the target cell (Herberman & Holden, 1978). This characteristic of spontaneous cytotoxicity makes the natural killer cell an important first line of defense against cancer and viral infections. Evidence that natural killer cells are protective against malignancy is found in studies of patients with large tumors who exhibit reduced levels of natural killer cell function (Herberman & Holden, 1978). Also, people and animals born without natural killer cells exhibit dramatically increased incidences of malignancies (Herberman & Holden, 1978).

Since patients with Down syndrome experience increased risks of infections and leukemia, it is possible that they are deficient in natural killer cell function. However, normal natural killer cell activity has been found in patients with Down syndrome (Noble & Warren, 1987b) which agrees with several earlier studies (Nurmi et al., 1982; Spina, Smith, Korn, Fahey, & Grossman, 1981), but contrasts with another (Matheson, Green, & Tan, 1981).

Autoimmunity in Down Syndrome

Patients with Down syndrome and their mothers also are believed to have an increased frequency of autoantibodies against thyroid antigens (Burgio et al., 1965). This is a most interesting finding because it associates Down syndrome with an autoimmune phenomenon. However, the clinical relevance of autoantibodies reactive to thyroid tissue in Down syndrome is not clear because these antibodies do not appear to be associated with a deficiency or pathological change in the thyroid.

Australia Antigen in Down Syndrome

Australia antigen is a surface antigen of the hepatitis B virus which causes type B acute hepatitis (Prince, 1968). When people become infected with the hepatitis B virus, the Australia antigen can be found in their blood (Bayer, Blumberg, & Werner, 1968). If a person has this antigen in the blood but does not have active hepatitis or jaundice, he or she is said to be a

◆

"carrier" of the Australian antigen. Studies have found that patients with Down syndrome are more frequently carriers of the Australia antigen than subjects without Down syndrome (Bayer et al., 1968; Stutnick, London, Blumberg, & Gerstley, 1972). This increased incidence of the Australia antigen resulting from infection of type B virus casts further suspicion on the integrity of the immune system in Down syndrome.

PROSPECTS FOR IMPROVING IMMUNE FUNCTION IN DOWN SYNDROME

The author and his colleagues are attempting to identify agents that will restore or instill immune competence in the patient with Down syndrome. A compound called PR 879–317A has recently been described that enhances the activity of peripheral blood mononuclear cells from patients with Down syndrome following treatment of these cells in this compound in test tubes (1 percent) (Warren, Healey, Johnston, Sidwell, Radov, Murray, & Kinsolving, 1987). Also, efforts are under way throughout the world to produce other substances to improve the immune functions of cancer patients, transplant recipients, and people with the Acquired Immunodeficiency Syndrome (AIDS). Perhaps people with Down syndrome will benefit from such efforts.

REFERENCES

Bayer, M.E., Blumberg, B.S., & Werner, B. (1968). Particles associated with Australia antigen in the sera of patients with leukemic, Down syndrome, and hepatitis. *Nature, 218,* 1057.

Benda, C.E., & Strassmann, G.S. (1965). The thymus in mongolism. *Journal of Mental Deficiency Research, 9*(2), 109.

Burgio, G.R., Severi, F., Rossoni, R., & Vaccaro, R. (1965). Mongolism and thyroid autoimmunity. *Lancet, 1,* 166.

Deaton, J.G. (1973). The mortality rate and causes of death among institutionalized monguls in Texas. *Journal of Mental Deficiency Research, 17,* 117.

Herberman, R.B., & Holden, T. (1978). Natural cell-mediated immunity. In G. Klein & S. Weinhouse (Eds.), *Advances in cancer research* (Vol. 27, p. 305). New York: Academic Press.

Levin, S. (1979). The immune system in Down syndrome. *Down's Syndrome, 1,* 2.

Levin, S., Schlesinger, M., Handzel, A., Hahn, T., Altman, Y., Czernobilsky, B., & Boss, J. (1979). Thymic deficiency in Down's syndrome. *Pediatrics, 63,* 80.

Matheson, D.S., Green, B., & Tan, H.Y. (1981). Human interferons alpha and beta inhibit T-cell dependent and stimulate T-cell independent mitogenesis and natural cytotoxicity: Relationship to chromosome 21. *Cellular Immunology, 65,* 366.

Noble, R.L., & Warren, R.P. (1987a). Altered T-cell subsets and defective T-cell function in young children with Down syndrome. *Immunological Communications* (in press).

Noble, R.L., & Warren, R.P. (1987b). Analysis of blood cell populations, plasma zinc, and natural killer cell activity in young children with Down syndrome. *Journal of Mental Deficiency Research* (in press).

Nurmi, T., Muttanen, K., Lassila, O., Henttonen, M., Sakkinen, A., Linna, S., & Tillikainen, A. (1982). Natural killer cell function in trisomy-21 (Down's syndrome). *Clinical and Experimental Immunology, 47*, 735.

Prince, A.M. (1968). An antigen detected in the blood during the incubation period of severe hepatitis. *Proceedings of the National Academy of Science, 60*, 814.

Scoll, T., Stein, A., & Hansen, H. (1982). Leukemia and other cancers, anomalies, and infections as causes of death in Down's syndrome in the United States during 1976. *Developmental Medicine and Child Immunology, 24*, 817.

Spina, C.A., Smith, D., Korn, E., Fahey, J.L., & Grossman, H.J. (1981). Altered cellular immune functions in patients with Down's syndrome. *American Journal of Diseases of Children, 131*, 251.

Stutnick, A.I., London, W.T., Blumberg, B.S., & Gerstley, B.J.S. (1972). Persistent anicteric hepatitis with Australian antigen in patients with Down's syndrome. *American Journal of Clinical Pathology, 57*, 2.

Szigeti, R., Revesz, T., & Schuler, D. (1974). Cell-mediated immune response in patients with Down's syndrome. *Acta Pediatric Academy of Science (Hungary), 15*, 31.

Warren, R.P., Healey, M.C., Johnston, A.V., Sidwell, R.W., Radov, L.A., Murray, R.J., & Kinsolving, C.R. (1987). Incubation in PR 879–317A enhances in vitro immune activity of peripheral blood mononuclear cells from patients with Down syndrome. *International Journal of Immunopharmacology* (in press).

Whittingham, S., Pitt, D.B., Sharma, D.L.B., & MacKay, I.R. (1977). Stress deficiency of the T-lymphocyte system exemplified by Down syndrome. *Lancet, 1*, 163.

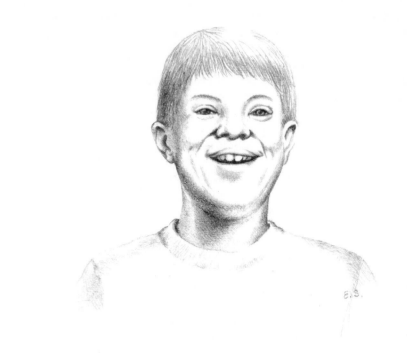

CHAPTER THREE
MEDICAL CONSIDERATION

J. DENNIS ODELL

The life expectancy and quality of life for individuals with Down syndrome has improved dramatically over the past 50 years. In 1929, the average life expectancy was only 9 years, and in 1961 it was 18.3 years (Thase, 1982). With changing attitudes in caring for the handicapped, the availability of improved medical technology, and greater awareness of health problems associated with Down syndrome, many individuals with Down syndrome are living well into adulthood. At all ages, however, caring for those with Down syndrome is a tremendous challenge.

Individuals with Down syndrome and their families require the services of many different health professionals. In addition, awareness of services available in the community for early intervention, education, and vocational training is vital. In some communities, there are multispecialty clinics available specifically for those with Down syndrome. In most communities, however, medical expertise is available but without programs specifically directed toward the handicapped. Oftentimes, health care is suboptimal because of incomplete knowledge of the many-faceted disorder and failure to coordinate services. In all communities, therefore, it seems that the best approach is for the family to utilize a family physician or pediatrician who has a knowledge of the issues involved in the health care of those with Down syndrome. This physician can provide the routine health services including well-child care, immunizations, and screening tests, helping the family make decisions regarding education and vocation, and coordinating the services of all the health care specialists who will need to be involved in the health care program. Optimal health care management requires a patient advocate who can help the family make the best use of the health care system; this service can best be provided by the family physician or pediatrician.

The following is a review of the health problems that are most commonly seen in Down syndrome, along with recommended screening measures to detect these problems. The recommendations will undoubtedly change as health care for individuals with Down syndrome becomes even more sophisticated, but the information should still help the family and physician develop a program for optimizing health care for patients with Down syndrome.

CONGENITAL HEART DISEASE

Congenital heart disease is the most common potentially serious health problem seen in Down syndrome. Cardiac malformations are found in about 40 percent of newborns (Spicer, 1984). Heart disease is the major contributor to the higher mortality rate seen in infants with Down syndrome in the first 2 years of life.

Many types of cardiac defects can be seen in Down syndrome, but the two most common are endocardial cushion defects (36 percent) and ventricular septal defects (33 percent). The endocardial cushions are ridges in the developing fetal heart that are involved in the formation of the septum that separates the right and left atria, part of the septum that separates right and left ventricles, and of the two valves between the atria and ventricles. Defects in the formation of these structures leads to complete or partial atrioventricular canals (Fig. 3-1). In the most common type seen in Down syndrome (complete atrioventricular canal), the defect leads to abnormal communication between the two atria, between the two ventricles, and one large abnormal valve separating the atria and ventricles instead of the normal two.

The symptoms of complete atrioventricular canal are a result of the large increase of blood flow into the lungs and of the abnormal function of the common atrioventricular valve. Severe heart failure, frequent pneumonia, and poor growth are frequently the result. Signs that may be seen are poor feeding, poor weight gain, easy fatigability, excessive sweating, duskiness, and shortness of breath. These are usually seen in early infancy.

The other common defect, ventricular septal defect, is an abnormal communication between the right and left ventricles. The symptoms depend on the size of the defect and can range from no symptoms in small defects to symptoms as severe as those due to atrioventricular canals.

Pulmonary artery hypertension is also frequently seen in Down syndrome. This is a constriction of the blood vessels in the lungs, causing back pressure and overload on the right ventricle. This is often a consequence of the increased flow to the lungs caused by the heart defects. It can also be seen without associated heart anomalies; in these cases, it is presumably a consequence of obstruction of the upper airways, which can occur in Down syndrome from the tongue, tonsils, and adenoids.

Because the dynamics of the heart change so dramatically during the first few weeks of life, the signs of severe congenital heart disease may not be apparent at birth. For optimal management, it is imperative that cardiac defects be diagnosed as early as possible. For this reason, in addition to a thorough physical examination in the neonatal period, an electrocardiogram, a chest x-ray, and possibly an echocardiogram are recommended for all newborns with Down syndrome, even those without symptoms (Spicer, 1984). Almost always, severe abnormalities of the heart will be detected in this way.

There are many other cardiac abnormalities that occur more frequently in Down syndrome, and in approximately 30 percent of those with heart defects, there are multiple abnormalities. Treatment depends on the severity of the symptoms. Conservative treatment of heart failure includes restricting fluid intake and the use of digitalis and diuretics. If symptoms become unmanageable, then surgery is warranted. Although surgical mortality is high (10–30%), improved technology and newer approaches

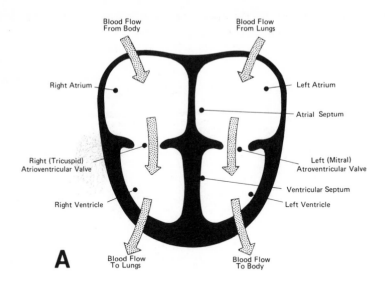

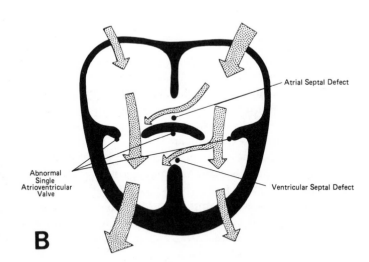

Figure 3–1. Schematic diagrams comparing the blood flow of (A) a normal heart, with equal amounts of blood entering and leaving both sides, and (B) a heart with complete atrioventricular canal with an atrial septal defect, a ventricular septal defect, and an abnormal atrioventricular valve. Because pressures on the left side of the heart are greater than the right, some blood is shunted from left to right across the septal defects, resulting in an increased flow to the lungs and an overload on the heart.

to surgical management have markedly improved the outcome in infants with congenital heart disease.

GASTROINTESTINAL DISORDERS

Gastrointestinal malformations are seen commonly in Down syndrome with an overall incidence of about 12 percent (Knox & Benzel, 1972). Many of these malformations can be life threatening unless detected early and surgically corrected. Anomalies can be seen in virtually any area of the gastrointestinal tract, but several are seen most commonly. These include tracheoesophageal fistula, pyloric stenosis, duodenal atresia, annular pancreas, imperforate anus, and Hirschsprungs' Disease.

Tracheoesophageal fistula is an anomaly involving an abnormal communication between the trachea and esophagus. There are many different types, each of differing severity, but all cause ingested substances to be aspirated into the lungs. Treatment in all cases is surgical.

Pyloric stenosis is a constriction of the outlet of the stomach that prevents passage of food from the stomach to the small intestine. Infants with pyloric stenosis have projectile vomiting and are usually ravenously hungry. Symptoms usually present at 1–2 months of age. Diagnosis is usually apparent based on clinical symptoms and can be confirmed by x-ray examination of the stomach after the child has swallowed barium.

Duodenal atresia is a malformation in which the duodenum is obstructed. An annular pancreas involves a pancreas that surrounds the duodenum and constricts the lumen, leading to duodenal obstruction. These lesions are present at birth, and symptoms are seen as soon as the newborn is fed. Vomiting is again the cardinal feature, but in these lesions it is usually bilious. Bilious vomiting in any newborn with Down syndrome should be considered due to a duodenal obstruction until proven otherwise. Diagnosis can usually be made by an abdominal x-ray.

Imperforate anus is an absence of the anal opening and diagnosis is made at the time of the newborn exam. Hirschsprungs' disease can be difficult to diagnose. It involves an absence of the nerve cells in the rectum and colon that stimulate intestinal motility, and the major symptom is severe constipation but usually with soft stools.

Duodenal obstruction, and some types of tracheoesophageal fistulas, can be suspected prenatally because they usually lead to an abnormally large volume of amniotic fluid; they may be detected by prenatal ultrasound. In all cases, treatment is surgical, and outcome is usually favorable if detected early.

Older individuals with Down syndrome may also have gastrointestinal disturbances. Occasionally, intestinal obstructive lesions may be incomplete and may not become apparent until an older age. Symptoms will usually include intermittent vomiting and poor growth. Another area of concern is malabsorption of intestinal contents. The extent of the problem is not yet clear, but there have been multiple reports of incomplete absorption of certain vitamins, minerals, and food. Studies have led to conflicting results, however, and delineation of the problem awaits further research.

ORTHOPEDIC PROBLEMS

Most of the orthopedic difficulties found in Down syndrome are not congenital anomalies but rather a consequence of the generally low muscle tone. The orthopedic disorder that has received the most attention recently is atlantoaxial subluxation (cervical spine instability). General awareness of the problem came about initially in 1983 because of a requirement that all persons with Down syndrome who wanted to participate in Special Olympics be screened for atlantoaxial subluxation prior to participation. There was concern that even mild trauma to the neck in an individual with an unstable cervical spine could lead to severe spinal injury. In fact, this has happened rarely, in spite of the fact that instability occurs in 10–20 percent of individuals with Down syndrome (Antony, 1986).

Atlantoaxial subluxation is an abnormal increase in mobility within the joint between the first two cervical vertebrae in the neck. The cause is unclear, but it is probably related to ligament laxity and abnormalities of the vertebrae themselves. Most children with Down syndrome who have x-ray evidence of instability have no symptoms. If symptoms are present, they are related to spinal cord compression—neck pain, change in gait pattern, weakness in extremities, spasticity, limited neck movement, and bowel or bladder incontinence. Diagnosis is made by taking side-view x-rays of the neck when the neck is fully flexed and fully extended so that abnormal instability can be detected.

If instability is present and there are no symptoms, restricting the individual from high-risk activities is probably sufficient intervention. These activities include any activities that could put significant stress on the neck, such as high jumping, diving, gymnastics, trampoline, and butterfly strokes in swimming (Lawhon). If symptoms are present, surgery is recommended and involves fusion of the joint. Because there are usually no symptoms, and consequences are potentially severe, it is recommended that all children with Down syndrome over 2 years of age and symptomatic individuals at any age be screened for atlantoaxial subluxation by x-ray (Pueschel, 1987).

Other orthopedic defects have received less attention but may cause difficulty for the individual with Down syndrome. Scoliosis (curvature of the spine) is seen frequently, but it is usually mild. Rarely is orthopedic intervention required, but if scoliosis is detected, periodic reevaluation needs to be done to ensure that there is no progression of the curvature or development of symptoms.

Dislocation of the hips has been reported to be more common in Down syndrome than in the normal population. This is probably due to the laxity of the tissues around the hip joint. This is a disabling condition that leads to marked limitation in walking. Degeneration of the hip joint and knee instability are also relatively common in Down syndrome. Foot problems, including flat feet and forefoot abnormalities are very common in individuals with Down syndrome and if left untreated can lead to significant disability (Diamond, Lynne, & Sigman, 1981). Because there may be no complaints until symptoms are severe, foot disorders can be easily overlooked. All of these orthopedic problems should be looked for in each routine well care visit.

GROWTH AND DEVELOPMENT

Maintaining good health and nutrition is vital for optimal mental and physical health in children with Down syndrome. Many of the congenital and acquired defects that are present in Down syndrome adversely affect growth and development, but even without other anomalies, growth rates and ultimate size are lower in Down syndrome. At birth, most full-term newborns with Down syndrome have lower lengths and weights than those without Down syndrome, and prematurity is not uncommon. Head circumference may be normal at birth. During the first 3 years of life, the growth velocity is slower than in the general population, so that by 3 years of age height is usually well below average. Adult height also is usually well below average (Cronk, 1978). The rate of weight gain is also slower than average, but not as slow as height velocity. Weight gain is especially slow in those with congenital heart disease. The growth in head size is also slower and usually follows the same pattern as height. When matched for height, rather than age, head circumference is usually in the low-average range compared with the general population. Growth charts are available for children with Down syndrome (see Appendix on page 199) and are useful in identifying those with abnormal growth patterns. Growth charts that are used for the general population will not be as helpful, because even healthy children with Down syndrome will rarely fall within the normal range (Cronk, Chumela, & Roche, 1985).

Attention to good nutrition is important at all ages. Maintaining an optimal growth pattern is the best proof of adequate nutrition. Obesity is a common problem and may be apparent as early as 2 or 3 years of age. Weight should be followed using standard weight-for-stature charts rather than standard weight-for-age curves (Cronk et al., 1985). Estimates for caloric requirements should also be based on height rather than age and may be lower if activity levels are low. Maintaining an adequate caloric intake, a balanced diet, and physical exercise are as important in those with Down syndrome as they are for the general population. It is not yet clear if vitamins and mineral requirements are higher in Down syndrome. Normal levels of vitamin supplements are certainly appropriate, but high vitamin doses may be harmful and should be avoided unless further research demonstrates definite benefits.

The age at which primary and secondary teeth erupt is usually delayed in Down syndrome, and tooth anomalies are not uncommon. Periodontal disease has been reported to be common, especially in those people with Down syndrome residing in institutions. Regular dental checkups and hygiene are important to prevent dental problems in those with Down syndrome (Pueschel et al., 1987).

Pubertal changes also are usually delayed in adolescents with Down syndrome. The average age for onset of menstruation is about 12.5 years, which is half a year delayed compared with the general population. Ovulation patterns are probably normal in most women with Down syndrome and pregnancies have occurred. In males, development of secondary sex characteristics is also delayed slightly, but the sequence of development is normal, and the changes in hormone levels normally seen in puberty are present. Masturbation is common in both sexes. Males are probably infertile, but this issue has not been settled for certain (Pueschel et al., 1987).

Thyroid disorders are common in Down syndrome. In older individuals with Down syndrome, as many as 50 percent may have thyroid abnormalities, usually hypothyroidism (Pueschel et al., 1987). The symptoms of hypothyroidism are delayed growth and short stature, obesity, lethargy, and dry skin. Because these symptoms mimic the normal appearance of individuals with Down syndrome, the possibility of hypothyroidism may be overlooked. For this reason, routine periodic screening for thyroid disorders is recommended in all persons with Down syndrome. Congenital hypothyroidism is about 30 times more common than usual in newborns with Down syndrome (Fort et al., 1984). Most states routinely screen all neonates for hypothyroidism, but if this is not done, thyroid tests should be done in newborns with Down syndrome.

HEARING IMPAIRMENT

Hearing impairments are frequent in Down syndrome, being seen in as many as 75 percent of cases (Schultz and Pueschel, 1984). Usually, hearing loss is mild to moderate in degree, and it is most often due to persistent fluid in the middle ear. The middle ear is located behind the ear drum and functions as a transformer of sound from the ear drum to the inner ear where the sound is converted to nerve impulses. When fluid instead of air is present in the middle ear cavity, the efficiency of sound transmission is decreased, and hearing loss results. Normally, the eustachian tube provides an opening between the middle ear and the throat and allows for drainage, but it if becomes blocked, fluid accumulation in the middle ear results. Persistent middle ear effusion is common in Down syndrome, presumably because of obstruction of the eustachian tubes by the tongue and adenoids and because of laxity of the walls of the eustachian tubes.

Ear infections are also extremely common in Down syndrome. Middle ear effusion predisposes one to ear infections, and impaired immune functioning may also contribute to the increased incidence of ear infections.

Aggressive treatment of ear infections, middle ear effusions, and hearing loss is imperative in children with Down syndrome, as acquisition of speech and communication will be hindered without correctly functioning ears. Diagnosis of ear infections is difficult in children with Down syndrome because the external ear canals are often very narrow, making visualization of the ear drum sometimes impossible. Wax accumulation is common, compounding the problem. Ear problems should be suspected in any child with chronic nasal congestion. If aggressive use of antibiotics, including long-term therapy, fails to alleviate the problem, placement of ventilation tubes in the eardrums to drain the middle ear, and possibly adenoidectomy, is warranted. A wait-and-see approach in hopes that the child will grow out of the problem is usually not appropriate, as the consequences of hearing loss during the early years of life are too great. If surgery is undertaken, care should be taken to screen for atlantoaxial instability first because intubation and surgery on tonsils or adenoids can stress the cervical spine.

ALZHEIMER'S DISEASE AND SEIZURES

Alzheimer's Disease is a disorder that causes presenile, dementia with memory loss and mental deterioration, usually in middle-aged and elderly people. There is a familial predisposition to the disease, and the cause is at present unknown, although there is some evidence that the abnormality that causes Alzheimer's Disease is due to a defective gene located on chromosome 21. The anatomical changes of Alzheimer's Disease appears to be almost universal in adults with Down syndrome over the age of 35 (Wisniewski et al., 1985). In spite of the anatomic findings of Alzheimer's Disease in adults with Down syndrome, most will show no signs of the disease. Early stages of Alzheimer's Disease are loss of advanced cognitive ability, which would not be evident in those with mental retardation. In those with Down syndrome, more advanced disease will be manifested as personality changes, withdrawal, incontinence, deterioration in mental performance, and possibly convulsions.

In an adult with Down syndrome, personality changes and mental deterioration may be due to Alzheimer's Disease, but there are many other correctable problems common to Down syndrome that could lead to the same symptoms. Cataracts, thyroid dysfunction, hearing loss, and other health problems should be ruled out before it is assumed changes are caused by Alzheimer's Disease.

Seizures and Other Conditions

Seizure activity is seen in infants and young children with Down syndrome about as frequently as in the general population. Beginning at age 20 to 30, however, grand mal seizures are seen more frequently in people with Down syndrome. This increased incidence in adulthood is probably due to stroke or other conditions usually seen in older populations (Madsen, 1987).

OPHTHALMOLOGICAL DISORDERS

A variety of disorders of the eye are found more frequently in people with Down syndrome than in the general population and are important to look for in all age groups (Peterson, 1984). Cataracts can be seen in infancy and are seen in most adults. The majority of cataracts are not significant enough to affect vision and rarely require surgery. Strabismus is frequent. If strabismus persists, loss of vision in one eye can result, so early detection and treatment are imperative. Refractive errors are seen in as many as 80 percent, usually due to myopia. An uncommon but potentially severe complication in Down syndrome is keratoconus. Keratoconus is a thinning and abnormal bulging of the cornea. It usually first appears during puberty, and initial symptoms are usually a reduction in vision. Acute relapses may occur, characterized by pain, redness, tearing, and cloudiness of the cornea, which may be followed by blindness (Walsh, 1981). Since the individual with Down syndrome will rarely complain of symptoms in any of these disorders, a search for eye problems must be included in routine screening examinations, and periodic evaluation by an ophthalmologist is recommended.

INFECTIOUS DISEASE AND MALIGNANCY

The incidence of pneumonia and other infectious diseases is strikingly high in Down syndrome, especially in early infancy and late adulthood (Thase, 1982). Despite tremendous advances in treatment with antibiotics and early recognition of disease, these diseases are still a major cause of morbidity and premature mortality in children and adults with Down syndrome. Much of the increased incidence in childhood is due to the increased number of infections seen in those with congenital heart disease. Without heart disease, the risk in children is certainly much lower. Still, however, respiratory illnesses and ear, nose, and throat infections appear to be very frequent occurrences in children with Down syndrome.

There are several factors leading to the higher infection rate. First, associated complications such as heart disease, pulmonary hypertension, nutritional problems, and any general debilitated state will predispose toward more infection. In adults who are nonambulatory, there is a twofold higher mortality risk from pneumonia as compared with ambulatory persons. Therefore, optimal management of other complications is helpful in keeping the rate of infections down. Second, there is much evidence that there is depressed immune function in persons with Down syndrome (see Chapter 2). In adults with Down syndrome, it appears that immune functioning deteriorates with increasing age, which would contribute to the frequent health problems seen in those over 40. Third, persons with Down syndrome are oftentimes more frequently exposed to infectious diseases than others. In childhood, involvement in early intervention programs and day care exposes children with Down syndrome to other children and the various diseases that children tend to carry. Many adults with Down syndrome are in institutions that often serve as reservoirs for infectious diseases, and epidemics are not uncommon. For this reason, preventative measures such as influenza, pneumococcal, and Haemophilus Influenza B vaccinations are important in keeping infection rates down in these settings.

The incidence of most types of cancer is probably normal or subnormal in Down syndrome, but leukemia is seen 15–30 times as often in children with Down syndrome than in the general population and is also seen more commonly in adults (Scholl et al., 1982). Leukemia can often be suspected based on clinical grounds and simple lab tests, but definitive diagnosis requires bone marrow examination. In the past, leukemia had a universally poor outcome, but long-term cure rates are now in the neighborhood of 50–60 percent of those afflicted. Early detection improves prognosis, so even without symptoms, periodic blood counts may be warranted.

SUMMARY

The life expectancy for a newborn with Down syndrome is now approximately 35–40 years, and for those that survive to age 10, life expectancy is greater than 45 years (Thase, 1982). Much can yet be done to improve life expectancy and the degree of health by anticipating possible health problems and preventing complications whenever possible.

In the neonatal period, a thorough search should be made for congenital defects, especially congenital heart disease, gastrointestinal anomalies, cataracts, and orthopedic disorders. Laboratory studies should include chromosome karyotyping, thyroid screening, electrocardiogram, and chest x-ray.

Throughout infancy, childhood, adolescence, and adulthood, periodic health maintenance evaluations are essential. Routine vaccinations should be given, and nonroutine immunizations such as pneumococcal and influenza vaccines should be considered. Close monitoring of growth using growth charts for children with Down syndrome and weight-for-stature charts in older individuals helps to assess for adequate nutrition. Potential obesity needs to be anticipated and prevented.

Thorough history and physical examination helps to detect complications as they arise. Screening tests should also include periodic thyroid function tests, blood counts, and hearing and vision testing. Examination by a pediatric cardiologist and ophthalmologist is appropriate during early childhood. Neck x-rays should be taken at age 2 and whenever symptoms suggestive of cervical spine instability are present. The periods of greatest risk for serious disease are childhood, with its high risks for congenital heart disease, gastrointestinal anomalies, infection, and leukemia, and late adulthood, with its high risks for pneumonia and Alzheimer's disease.

Providing good health programs for those with Down syndrome is a challenging undertaking for health care professionals. Knowledge of the general problems that can occur, awareness of the services available in the community, and a good working relationship with the individual with Down syndrome, the family, and all involved in providing health care needs are required for the best health maintenance program.

The purpose of this chapter has been to draw attention to specific medical needs of people who have Down syndrome and to suggest that the physician and family pay particular attention to the possibility of need for extra care in these areas. It is assumed that other routine areas would be examined, just as with other people. The interrelationship between physical and mental health for individuals with Down syndrome is much the same as for the general population and mental health concerns are similar.

ACKNOWLEDGMENT

The author appreciates the assistance of Allen Crocker, M.D., Boston Children's Hospital, in reviewing this chapter.

REFERENCES

Antony, R.M. (1986). Alantoaxial instability: Why the sudden concern? *Adapted Physical Activity Quarterly, 3,* 320–328.
Cronk, C.E. (1978). Growth of children with Down syndrome: Birth to age 3 years. *Pediatrics, 61,* 564–568.
Cronk, C.E., Chumela, W.C., & Roche, A.F. (1985). Assessment of overweight children with trisomy 21. *American Journal of Mental Deficiency, 89,* 433–436.
Diamond, L.S., Lynne, D., & Sigman, B. (1981). Orthopedic disorders in patients with Down syndrome. *Orthopedic Clinics of North America, 12,* 57–71.
Fort, P., Lifshiz, F., Bellisario, R., Davis, J., Lanes, R., Pugliese, M., Richman, R., Post, E.M., & David, R. (1984). Abnormalities of thyroid function in infants with Down syndrome. *The Journal of Pediatrics, 104,* 545–549.
Knox, G.E. & Benzel, R.W. (1972). Gastrointestinal malformations in Down syndrome. *Minnesota Medicine, 55,* 542–544.
Lawhon, S.M. Atlantoaxial instability in Down syndrome: Guidelines for screening. Cincinnati, OH: Orthopaedic Consultants of Cincinnati.
Madsen, J. (1987). Personal communication, July 8, 1987.
Peterson, R.A. (1984). Ophthalmological manifestations. In S.M. Pueschel (Ed.), *The young child with Down syndrome.* New York: Human Science Press.
Pueschel, S.M. (1984). *The young child with Down syndrome.* New York: Human Science Press.
Pueschel, S.M., Tingey, C., Rynders, J.E., Crocker, A.C., & Cutcher, D.M. (Eds.). (1987). *New perspectives on Down syndrome.* Baltimore: Brookes.
Scholl, T., Stein, Z., & Hansen, H. (1982). Leukemia and other cancers, anomalies and infections as causes of death in Down's syndrome in the United States during 1976. *Developmental Medicine and Child Neurology, 24,* 817–829.
Shultz, M.C., and Pueschel, S.M. (1984). Audiological assessments. In S.M. Pueschel (Ed.), *The young child with Down syndrome.* New York: Human Science Press.
Spicer, R.L. (1984). Cardiovascular disease in Down syndrome. *Pediatric Clinics of North America, 31,* 1331–1343.
Thase, M.E. (1982). Longevity and mortality in Down syndrome. *Journal of Mental Deficiency Research, 26,* 177–192.
Update: The 1987 preventive medicine checklist for Down's syndrome individuals of all ages. (1987). *Down's Syndrome Papers and Abstracts for Professionals,* pp. 2–7.
Walsh, S.Z. (1981). Keratoconus and blindness in 469 institutionalized subjects with Down syndrome and other causes of mental retardation. *Journal of Mental Deficiency Research, 25,* 243–251.
Wisniewski, K.E., Wisniewski, H.M., & Wen, G.Y. (1985). Occurrence of neuropathological changes and dementia of Alzheimer's Disease in Down's syndrome. *Annals of Neurology, 17,* 278–282.

PART TWO

FAMILY

No one plans to have a handicapped child. Although some parents of children with Down syndrome may have had prenatal diagnoses and thus are already aware of the child's sex and condition, most parents learn of the child's condition the day the baby is born, or shortly after. Most families begin the pregnancy with the hope and expectation that this child will be the child they always wanted, someone who will be able to do all the things that they wanted to do and then some. Finding that the child has a handicap is a shock to the entire family. Perhaps it is more of a shock to families of children with Down syndrome, since the news usually comes before the mother and father have been able to rest from the exhausting excitement of the delivery.

The initial shock experienced by parents is followed by many questions, among them, "Why did this happen?" or "why did this happen to me?" Thus begins an ongoing need for comfort and information. Many parents find it helpful to meet other parents of children with Down syndrome. This, along with genetic counseling, can help parents to cope with their child's condition.

New parents of children with Down syndrome also may find support in their own parents. Grandparents are aware of the intrinsic joys of parenting, but are also concerned for the demands and strains their own adult children will experience. They will also have to adjust to the knowledge that their grandchild, whose birth they proudly awaited, will not be the child they expected.

Siblings of children with Down syndrome will also be presented with challenges they would not normally face. Older children are frequently expected to share in the child-rearing responsibilities, and younger siblings are in the unusual situation of becoming, at some time in their lives, "older" than their chronologically older brother or sister. Although it is important for parents to provide special care for their child with Down syndrome, it is equally important for them to remember the needs of their other children.

When a family has a handicapped child, there is always some disruption to the family circle. For some families the strain is so great that the circle is broken, for others, the circle becomes stronger.

This section covers the triad of family concerns presented above. First, Chapter 4 reviews the importance of counseling parents and families. Practical steps are recommended for working with the family of a child with Down syndrome. The reaction of parents and grandparents of children with Down syndrome is explored in Chapter 5. Finally, Chapter 6 presents a personal account of the younger sister of a child with Down syndrome.

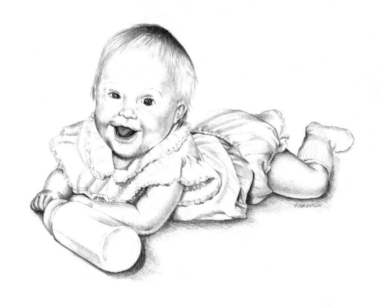

CHAPTER FOUR

COUNSELING THE FAMILY OF A CHILD WITH DOWN SYNDROME

JOHN C. CAREY AND CAROL TINGEY

♦

The experienced professional is in a vulnerable position when a child with Down syndrome is born. It becomes professionally necessary almost immediately to convey to the parents that there is something wrong. But most parents of newborns with Down syndrome who are not ill or in an intensive care nursery will not perceive their baby as "different" or having problems. The clues to the diagnosis in the newborn are subtle variations, not structurally obvious, and most new parents wouldn't recognize them. Infants with Down syndrome react and respond like most babies; thus, most parents will not feel anything different when they hold and care for the infant. They will not perceive that there is anything wrong with their infant, and therefore they will not be requesting information, help, or guidance.

Another unique aspect of the situation is that Down syndrome is one of the few common conditions in which the prediction of developmental disability can be made in the early days of life. This prediction is not based on the baby's own individual neurologic status or performance but is based on prior knowledge of the natural history of the developmental difficulties associated with Down syndrome. Thus, making a diagnosis based on the recognition of physical characteristics and predicting the child's future based on a chromosomal study will often seem vague, mysterious, and perhaps unrealistic to parents (Carey, 1982).

The relationship of the child's appearance to the child's functional ability is oversimplified. There is an automatic preconceived notion of the general public regarding the degree of developmental disability associated with Down syndrome. The high value in North American society on intelligence, its perceived relationship to importance, and the vague legal and social status of persons with retardation are all issues that enter into the meaning (and stigma) of Down syndrome. All of this comes with the diagnosis. No one can ever be completely prepared to enter the private world of the parents and give them this unwanted and usually unexpected information.

Down syndrome occurs in about 1 in 800–1,000 births. This prevalence figure makes the Down syndrome the most common condition diagnosed in the newborn period that has significant life impact. Because of the relatively common occurrence, professionals involved in the care of families need to be aware of current information regarding possible reactions of the parents and family in such a situation. Along with pleasant excitement, there is a crisis atmosphere that surrounds the birth of any child. The time of birth has its own unique set of psychological and social aspects. For the family of a child with Down syndrome, additional concerns are present.

Helping the family of a child with Down syndrome is a challenge for professionals and anyone who volunteers to help. Parents remember in great detail the events surrounding the initial discussions; they remember the kindness given to them by certain professionals and are continually hurt, even by the memory of insensitive experiences (see Chapter 5).

Being the bearer of less-than-good news is always a difficult task. Presenting a diagnosis or the result of an evaluation to families requires careful understanding of the condition of Down syndrome and of the possible reactions of parents. There are a number of approaches to counseling that may be helpful to the professional or parent who is in the position to help the family.

FAMILY REACTION TO THE BIRTH OF A CHILD WITH A CONGENITAL DEFECT: THE LITERATURE

Professionals from various disciplines have been interested in this complex topic. Discussion of the crisis of the birth of a child with a congenital defect and counseling approaches to this situation have been described from several perspectives (Table 4–1).

A number of authors have addressed the issue of reactions of parents to very specific problems. For example, there are several investigations that have attempted to study the feelings of parents who have had a child with Down syndrome. There are also works that have investigated reactions to other problems such as cleft lip, genital defects, and limb deficiency. Quite likely, there are specific aspects to the meaning of a particular problem, and there also may be the more general reactions that occur in anyone who has a newborn with an illness or abnormality. The differences in these meanings are probably related to the parents' values regarding children and, of course, to the meaning of life in the society and/or in the individual families.

Table 4–1.
Survey of Literature: Perspectives on Impact of the Birth of a Handicapped Child

Psychology of normal pregnancy
Family planning models
The meaning of a child to a family
Crisis intervention literature
Grief and mourning response literature
Parent-infant bonding
Fetal personhood
Psychoanalytic models and defense mechanisms
Genetic counseling
Adaptation in coping with stress
Specific studies on particular disorder (e.g., Down syndrome)

The two most crucial bodies of literature that have had some mention in this area involve the psychology of normal pregnancy and the meanings of a child in our society. Although information on both of these topics has been published, application to the birth of a child with a defect has received little discussion.

The reasons why human families have children are diverse and vary according to groups interviewed. Reasons for having children include (a) enhancing one's virility or femininity, (b) fulfilling biological destiny, (c) satisfying needs of one's own parents, (d) reaching toward immortality, (e) protection in old age, (f) a gift to one's parents, (g) fulfilling one's own aspirations, and, of course, (h) religious reasons. The impact on the family of the birth of a child with Down syndrome is related to the meaning or constellation of meanings that is unique to individual parents.

Models to Explain

It is possible to classify the last three decades of literature on the psychological aspects of the birth of the handicapped child into four theoretical models. The listing of these models helps emphasize the common psychological themes that have been stated over the years (Kessler, 1979).

The earliest approach to this topic was that of a psychoanalytic orientation. This model emphasized the defense mechanisms utilized by parents on finding out their child is handicapped. A review of this early literature implies a certain degree of pathology in the parents dealing with the birth of their child with a congenital defect (Irvin, Kennell, & Klaus, 1982).

The second model that one can abstract from the literature and that is recognized as a useful approach to the dilemma of parents is the grief for the lost child. This particular model indicates that the birth of a child with a congenital defect is similar to loss and grief. Parents are described as mourning the loss of their expected or fantasized child. This unique type of loss does seem to apply to parents in such a dilemma and is probably related to the psychology of normal pregnancy mentioned above (Myers, 1983).

The third model represents the orientation that has been labeled chronic sorrow. In this approach, the mourning and grief response surrounding loss is again emphasized, but the long-standing aspect to the sorrow is also stressed. More recent literature has emphasized that this aspect of chronic sorrow may not be a long-standing, stable level of reaction, but perhaps involves peaks and valleys occurring at certain milestones in the life of a handicapped child or at critical times in the family.

The fourth model could be labeled as an adaptation model or the development of coping strategies. This particular approach also emphasizes the similarity to grieving over a loss and describes the stages that parents go through at the birth of an infant with a congenital malformation (Irvin et al., 1982). Parents experience shock, denial, sadness–anger–anxiety, adaptation, and reorganization in various order and intensity. The terminology used here overlaps that in the literature on grief and crisis intervention and is not usually as familiar to pediatricians as to professionals in the behavioral sciences. This model suggests that parents are going through a dilemma, and most of their reactions are regarded as normal coping mechanisms rather than as implications of pathology, as in the psychoanalytic model. Thus, denial is usually a stage that is time-bound and is a practical "shock absorber" for the parents to gather the psychological strength with which to deal with the immediate and ongoing problems. This model implies a predictable course and gives the counselor a description of what the parents are going through in the situation.

Many authors who have dealt with the topic of the birth of a child with a defect have listed factors that are involved in the complex reactions of the parents to the situations. The variables involved, however, are so complicated that no single study is able to weigh their individual significance in any clear-cut fashion. Factors that probably affect the emotional involvement and reactions of parents at the time of birth include the following.

1. The individual personal adjustment of the parents to their role in parenthood is important. Even before they become parents, people have preconceived notions of what parenting means. These ideas grow and expand during pregnancy and as the family adjusts to having children in the home.
2. Demographic factors such as the education of parents, number of siblings, order of the child in the family, and parental age probably play some role in the emotional complex surrounding the birth. However, it is difficult from reading the literature to know in which direction these variables influence which reaction. Parents who have a first child with Down syndrome will state explicitly that they are glad that this was their first so that they could enjoy the child without making comparisons, while parents who have a child who is born later in the order will stress the benefits of the other children to help love and care for the child.
3. The community and cultural attitudes toward handicaps are important to parents. Various society and religious organizations place different values on intelligence and have different attitudes toward the stigma of certain problems. The study of anthropologic aspects of stigma and disability could enhance the understanding of how the family problems relate to the community and the society.

4. The social aspects of the individual defect are important to parents. For example, children with Down syndrome may be more of a challenge to highly educated families due to the value of intellect to the family and their associates.
5. The availability of services for care of the child's problem is always important.
6. The parents' experience and skill with dealing with crises and disappointments in the past are important.
7. The genetic aspects of the condition are important. Conditions that are inherited are more intrusive than those that are acquired or environmentally caused. Families who find that the child has trisomy 21 Down syndrome may react differently than those who may themselves be carriers and, therefore, sustain more risk for other children with Down syndrome to be born into the family.

Although it might be assumed that the more severe deficits would generate deeper problems, this is not always true. Severity is a very subjective impression, and the perception of parents may be much different from the perception of professionals. Some families whose child has a less serious and more treatable defect, such as a cleft lip or a single missing finger, often appear to have as involved a reaction as parents of a child with Down syndrome.

Telling a parent that a child's condition could have been worse is an approach that was commonly used in the past at the birth of a child with a handicap; this approach *never helps* parents validate their feelings and never provides consolation. Although parents themselves frequently come to the decision that things could have been worse and their situation is not so bad, it does not help to try to lead them to such a conclusion.

Recurrent Themes

In addition to the models and issues mentioned above, there exists a number of other themes that consistently recur in the recent literature. Many of these themes come from discussions with parents who have experienced the birth of a child with a congenital defect, and it is remarkable how similar some of these themes are, even among people who have never talked to one another.

One of the more important and common themes is the issue of the cause of the defect, the search for cause, and its relationship to the feelings of responsibility. The birth of a child with a congenital malformation can often produce a plight that enters the realm of religion and existential philosophy. The question of meaning recurs again and again as it has in the above discussions. The very common questions of "Why me?" or

"What has this event to do with my past life?" commonly occur. Lacking a clear-cut answer as to the cause of the child's problem is more difficult than having an answer, even if the answer implies one's own responsibility.

It is difficult to deal with uncertainty. For this reason, parents' feelings of responsibility should never be brushed aside; rather, they should be validated as natural. Concern is a common feeling and certainly needs to be recognized by any helper.

Parents of a child with Down syndrome often face a complex double bind. If negative feelings are expressed, then the parent risks being labeled as nonaccepting or rejecting of the child. If positive feelings are expressed, then professionals or others may label the response as reaction formation, denial, or sublimation. Either way, the parents seem to be in a "damned if you do, damned if you don't" situation. The positive and nonpathological nature of coping mechanisms needs recognition in this situation.

The issue of hope also emerges as a common theme. Some authors have discussed this issue in detail. Hope obviously ties into the dilemma of meaning and the significance, religious or otherwise, of the event. Hope has been described as a defense against despair, as an actual coping mechanism, and as a way and manner to help one move into action. It is more inclusive and has more depth than wishing.

This leads to a theme that has not been dealt with extensively in the literature: That parents and their support persons are actually in the process of attempting to balance three paradoxes or conflicts.

The first paradox, of the presence of the already-existing parental bond to the child versus the grief response, has been emphasized above. This particular "tightrope" is especially difficult to walk during the first few days of the child's life. The recognition of this tightrope by helpers will sometimes put perspective on the parent's plight.

Second is the continuum of prediction for the child's future. On one side, there is a very gloomy and pessimistic picture; on the other side, there is a completely positive picture. Helping parents find a balance on this continuum is a challenge for the professional helper.

The third tightrope walked during the actual counseling involves the conflict of the parents' desire to treat the child as normally as possible on one side versus the attempt to accept the situation on the other. Sometimes these two ends will present a conflict, and the recognition of this continuum sometimes gives perspective to the helper.

Although detailed discussion of all of the themes that surround this important challenge is beyond the scope of this chapter, it is important to recognize the most frequent themes. A number of other themes and issues are mentioned briefly below because of their interplay with the above points.

1. Although professionals and other parents who help the affected parents try to see themselves as separated from the situation, individual feelings of responsibility and personal attitudes enter into the setting. These may inhibit a natural and effective interaction with the family.
2. Asynchronous or differently timed reactions of the two parents is a common occurrence and also plays a role. This can be a particularly important problem if the parents are experiencing communicative or relationship problems. Mothers who are not maintaining a relationship with the child's father may choose not to attempt to inform him or his family.
3. The concern that parents have about the impact of Down syndrome on the rest of their family, including siblings of the child, is an important issue, and any helpers should review the current literature on this topic.
4. The issues of the questioning of self-esteem and feelings of shame or disgrace are also involved in this birth event.
5. Changes in role organization and situation and practical child care demands are also aspects that are part of the larger picture.

The discussion thus far has emphasized the themes, principles, and issues that exist in the vast number of papers and discussions that have dealt with this topic. It is important to note, however, that much that has been written about the birth of a child with Down syndrome (or other congenital problems) has been the experience of a few counselors and involves only a few individual cases in each particular paper.

Although the remainder of this chapter deals with some of the more practical aspects of helping and counseling the family, it is important to note that there exists no longitudinal, detailed investigation into the variables surrounding the birth of a child and the growth of the family that can help guide the professional in choosing appropriate counseling techniques or procedures.

COUNSELING PROCEDURE

Counseling needs of families can be divided into two general categories: (a) the early period consisting of the initial informing interview and subsequent early conversations, and (b) ongoing assistance.

The Early Period: Goals and Objectives of the Informing Interview

From the existing literature on the topic of the birth of a handicapped child and from numerous interviews with parents, it is apparent that families vividly remember the events surrounding the birth. The professional or other helper in this situation has the opportunity and challenge to support the parents in a way that is remembered for the rest of their lives. The goals in counseling the family near the time of the birth of a child with Down syndrome include the following.

1. Promotion of the already-existing bonding process of the parents and the child

2. Helping parents work through the natural grief response that has been outlined above

3. Helping the parents develop an adaptive concern and become an advocate for their child

4. Presenting accurate and up-to-date information

5. Helping the parents become acquainted with other parents of children with Down syndrome

These goals can be carried out by the performance of the following, more specific objectives.

1. Follow the recommendations mentioned in the literature regarding the informing of the parents of a child with Down syndrome. These include telling both parents together (if possible) as early as possible in a private place with a concerned, compassionate, and informed attitude.

2. Provide the opportunity and a nonjudgmental atmosphere for the parents to ventilate their feelings, both mixed and positive, and to receive professional validation that all the feelings are natural.

3. Humanize the situation by having the child present, holding the child, calling the child by name, referring to ''children with Down syndrome'' rather than Down's children, and listening to the parents and repeating and rephrasing what they say to be sure you understand. It is also helpful at this time to ask the new parents if they would like to have another parent come to talk to them.

4. Have the most current information on the Down syndrome as well as knowledge of resources for care.

The National Down Syndrome Congress is a valuable resource in this area. Professionals, parents, and interested others can receive written material and names of local parent organizations by contacting Natural Down Syndrome Congress, 1800 Dempster Street, Park Ridge, IL 60068-1146, (800) 232-NDSC.

Plan of Action for the Counselor

Initial contact is made as soon as possible, usually the day the child is born or the next day. Both parents are informed together, if possible, in a private, comfortable setting. Begin the discussion with the medical and developmental implications of Down syndrome. Explain the process for chromosomal analysis and ask for the parents' permission to perform the procedure. Tell the parents that you will return the next day to answer other questions and to report the results of the chromosome analysis if it is ready.

The second visit is begun by asking the parents if there is something they want to know or are wondering about. The second interview should be a time of listening and clarification. By the time of this interview, the results of the chromosome study may not have returned. Ask the parents if they have questions about the procedure.

The third interview could be 2–3 days after the first interview and would probably be the time in which the chromosomal results are presented. Reading material can be given at this time if it hasn't been given at an earlier interview. The biology of chromosomes can be explained in more detail, and the initiation of the genetic counseling process can occur.

During all of these interviews, some assessment as to how the parents are dealing with the above-mentioned paradoxes should occur. Having the infant present during these meetings is something that parents usually appreciate. There should be some plan for follow-up, either by phone in a few days or in person in 1–3 weeks. Home visits are helpful if resources are available for them to occur. Discussion of such options as infant development programs and parent support groups can also occur during these initial interviews, and referral, if appropriate, could be made at discharge or at the initial follow-up contact. The timing of follow-up after this initial plan depends on the individual parents and their adaptation.

This outline for initial care can be coordinated by a professional who is able to obtain the up-to-date resources regarding the biology and natural history of Down syndrome. Pediatricians, family practice doctors, and/or obstetricians who have experience in an informing interview and can obtain current information on Down syndrome are the appropriate professionals to carry out this model program. Geneticists who have been experienced in such situations can be utilized as resources but do not necessarily have to be the primary initial helpers. The National Down Syndrome Congress can be used as a resource at any time during the process.

What to Expect in the Initial Counseling

All of the general issues that have been mentioned thus far apply to helping the family at the time of the birth of a child with Down syndrome. It is of note that there have been only 13 studies that have actually looked into the specific aspects of the informing interview for the parents at the time of the birth of the child with Down syndrome. Review of these investigations indicate that parents who have a child with Down syndrome wish to be told of the diagnosis as soon as possible, with both parents together in a private setting, and informed in as direct, honest, and sympathetic a way as possible.

In addition, parents prefer to have "immediate and available access to services that provide accurate, comprehensive, and practical support and guidance" (Cunningham, Morgan, & McGuder, 1984). Studies have indicated that parents *do* want to be told when the clinical diagnosis of Down syndrome has been made by the medical practitioners. The common assumption that it is probably better to wait does not seem to be borne out by these investigations. In fact, those that would argue that the parents need time to "bond with their baby" ignore the observation that bonding to the infant has started to occur long before the birth of the child.

Although parents must come to grips with both bonding and grieving, most parents seem to balance this paradox and move along in their adaptation. Although suggestions for counseling are consistent, a study by Cunningham et al. (1984) indicates, however, that the suggestions are frequently not implemented.

It is recommended that individual hospitals develop a preplanned procedure for parents to be informed of the diagnosis using the above suggestions; parents should also receive close follow-up during the early weeks. Preplanned procedures could be organized in hospitals where births occur and where the hospital would expect at least one infant with Down syndrome each year. Hospitals that have fewer than 800–1,000 births per year can rely on other resources in their community to provide services to families.

Any preplanned service or program should include the resources necessary to carry out the informing interview, the follow-up sessions, and genetic counseling (or referral for such a service), to make available current reading material for parents, and to offer referral to local parents of children with Down syndrome for support. Pediatricians are in the position of organizing and engineering such programs in their individual hospital settings. It is suggested that primary care physicians (pediatricians, family practitioners, or obstetricians) develop such a program by formally designating an experienced health care professional (e.g., a perinatal social worker, genetic counselor, or nurse-clinician) based at the hospital to be the program's consistent figure. This helping person can join with the physician in the informing sessions and assist in referral, follow-up, and acquisition of local resource information.

Other resources that are important to mention in this context include parent groups, both local or national. In addition to the structure of an organized parent group, hospitals and medical providers often know of particularly helpful parents who are willing to share their experiences with parents at the time of the birth. Even in communities where no local parent group is available, other parents who have worked through some of these feelings can be a model for the "new" parents. Books and pamphlets with current information regarding the disorder in question are important to obtain and have available for the family (Pueschel et al., 1980; Rynders & Harrobin, 1984).

Referral for genetic counseling is always an option for parents who have questions about the genetic and causal aspects of Down syndrome. Genetic counseling is not required for every family who has a child with Down syndrome, but it certainly should be considered when the professional is unable to answer the parents' questions or to find the resources to address the issues. Recurrence risk information regarding Down syndrome can be given to parents by their genetic counselor.

Other Considerations

Other issues that must constantly be kept in mind in the early counseling include the following.

1. Families can include a variety of parents, grandparents, close friends, babysitters, etc., and all are affected by socioeconomic status, religion, education, occupation, and income. These people may also need to talk to a counselor.

2. Having a child with Down syndrome is not a 9:00 A.M. to 5:00 P.M. job, but rather it is a lifelong task.

3. The normalcy of the family unit may be compromised or maximized depending on attitudes and services.

4. Parents may need help to see the child as a person and to remove the label of the diagnosis from the child.

5. Parents are going through a series of peaks and valleys. Do not expect them to accept the situation once and for all; rather, they will continually deal with old problems and have new concerns.

6. Parents can feel the discomfort the counselor feels and the projection of perceived inability to cope that the counselor may give.

7. Parents may need help to realize that family needs must supersede the child's needs and that no one person can be the focal point of the family.

8. Although parents need information, they do not need to have predictions as to the adult or life skills that the child will eventually have. Since these are at least partly determined by life experiences and training, they can not be accurately made even for nonhandicapped infants.

9. Most importantly, parents want understanding, but they do not want pity for themselves or for their child with Down syndrome.

Continuing Assistance

The ongoing assistance of the family is obviously as significant as the informing interview (Carey, 1987). At this particular time in the United States, infant programs provide much of the major support for parents of a child with Down syndrome. However, this does not exclude the fact that there may be other models and approaches to ongoing support. For example, a Salt Lake City physician has developed a parent support group in the setting of his own pediatric practice. In addition, pediatricians will often have infant educational specialists visit their office for consultation and involvement with children in their practice. Families often expect direction and ongoing support from the pediatrician. If the physician is trained in the psychodynamics of chronic illness and in the anticipatory guidance and well-child care model, and if the physician is interested, he or she can be of great comfort to the family. It is important for any professionals either to make the decision that they are going to commit to this ongoing support or to refer the infant and family to a service or setting that *can* help them with continuous support. Infant programs are often a service that provides this ongoing support; ideally, this can occur in conjunction with the medical care provider.

ASSISTANCE WITH DEVELOPMENTAL CONCERNS

Professionals recognize an immediate need to provide initial counseling and follow-up, and feelings of parents and professionals are strong during the early years. It is appropriate, therefore, to emphasize issues for parents and professionals in early counseling. It is, however, very short-sighted to assume that parents are only in need of help concerning issues related to the birth of the child. Perhaps because parents become occupied with the daily needs of the child after they take the child home, they have less opportunity to ask the scores of questions that they have concerning the child's developmental needs. Parents are also concerned about the problems related to adjusting household routines for all family members to meet the special needs of the child with Down syndrome (Tingey-Michaelis, 1983).

Parents continue to need assistance as the child grows, especially as the child is in need of new services (Michaelis, 1980; Tingey, 1987b) or as the child attempts to relate naturally to others in the family or community (Tingey, 1987a). Although, technically, parents could ask these questions tions of service providers, such providers may be inexperienced with few practical suggestions to offer. More information needs to be gathered concerning the needs of parents of children, teenagers, young adults, and adults with Down syndrome (Tingey, 1987). With this information, personnel and programs can be prepared to meet these needs.

CONCLUSIONS AND GENERAL RECOMMENDATIONS

As emphasized in this discussion, the person helping the family at the time of the birth of a child with a defect has unique opportunity and challenge. The available literature on this topic can assist the helping person in understanding the plight that is being experienced by the family. Although most of the experiences and written information is of a philosophical and case report nature, there are a number of practical themes and issues that have emerged and that have been reviewed here. The following might improve the setting and, therefore, the experience of the parents.

1. Programs to inform the public regarding handicapping conditions and their stigma, along with organized education of the general public regarding the genetic, causal, and biological aspects of Down syndrome and the uncertainty surrounding this condition due to the limitations of science.
2. Education of medical professionals regarding the feelings of parents, the principles of the informing interview, the availability of resources, and the natural history and biology of Down syndrome.
3. Prenatal visits by parents to the medical care providers for their child prior to birth.
4. Inclusion into childbirth classes of discussion of parents' fears and concerns about the possible birth of a child with a problem.
5. Availability in medical libraries and hospital settings of current information on Down syndrome and lists of local resources including parent groups.
6. In-place counseling procedures in all hospitals that have births.
7. In-place counseling procedures in all other facilities that may provide services to the growing child or to the family.

Even with all of these recommendations at their fullest, the birth of a child with Down syndrome will be a shock to the parents and extended family. However, the attitude and views of professionals and the general public can help reduce this pain.

ACKNOWLEDGEMENTS

The authors thank all the parents of children with Down syndrome who have shared with them and helped inform them. The authors also express thanks to Melanie Black and Joan Fitzgerald, M.S., for help in preparing this manuscript.

REFERENCES

Carey, J.C. (1982). Chromosome disorders. In A.M. Rudolph (Ed.), *Pediatrics* (pp. 242–247). Norwalk, CT: Appleton-Century-Croft.

Carey, J.C. (1987). Health supervision and anticipating guidance for infants with congenital defects. In R. Ballard (Ed.), *Care of the ICN graduate*. Philadelphia: Saunders.

Cunningham, C.C., Morgan, P.A., & McGuder, R.B. (1984). Down syndrome: Is dissatisfaction with disclosure of diagnosis inevitable? *Developmental Medicine Child Neurology, 26,* 33.

Irvin, N.A., Kennell, J.H., & Klaus, M.H. (1982). Caring for the parents of an infant with a congenital malformation. In M.H. Klaus & J.H. Kennell (Eds.), *Parent-infant bonding*. St. Louis: Mosby.

Kessler, S. (1979). *Genetic counseling: Psychological dimensions*. New York: Academic Press.

Michaelis, C.T. (1980). Things are worse now. *The Exceptional Parent, 10*(4), 29–42.

Myers, B.A. (1983). The informing interview. *American Journal of Diseases of Children, 137,* 574–577.

Pueschel, S.M., Canning, C.D., Murphy, A., & Zausmer, E. (1980). *Down syndrome: Growing and learning*. Kansas City, MO: Andrews and McMeel.

Rynders, J.E., & Horrobin, J.M. (1984). *To give an edge*. St. Paul, MN: Colwell.

Tingey-Michaelis, C. (1983). Repetition, relaxation routine. *The Exceptional Parent, 13*(3), 52–54.

Tingey, C. (1987a). Psychosocial development in persons with Down syndrome. In S. Pueschel, C. Tingey, J. Rynders, A. Crocker, & D. Crutcher (Eds), *New perspectives on Down syndrome*. Baltimore, MD: Brookes.

Tingey, C. (1987b). Cutting the umbilical cord: Parental perceptions. In S. Pueschel (Ed.), *The young person with Down syndrome: Transition from adolescence to adulthood*. Baltimore, MD: Brookes.

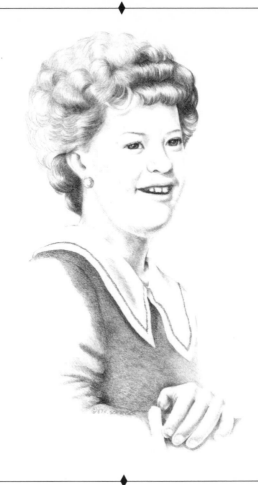

CHAPTER FIVE

PARENTS AND GRANDPARENTS OF CHILDREN WITH DOWN SYNDROME

DIANE CRUTCHER

◆

"I have a great life and a great family." So says Ashleigh Smith, a 13-year-old sixth-grade elementary school student, gymnast, artist, swimmer, and such an extrovert that her parents occasionally wish for a few moments of quiet. Ironically, it was the prospect of quiet that seemed a threat when Ashleigh was born.

Parents of children with Down syndrome face many of the same challenges that all parents have. There are, of course, nighttime feedings, daytime lunches, afternoon naps, and regular trips to the doctor. There are school clothes to get and birthday parties to give. In addition, there are many other lifelong challenges and problems unique to being the parent of a child with a handicap. These challenges cluster around the developmental needs of the child and the pressures and questions surrounding the day-to-day effort to meet those needs (Tables 5-1 and 5-2).

In order to understand how these challenges, pressures, and questions are woven into the parents' lives, let us consider the Smith family.

On November 11, 1973, a second daughter, Ashleigh, was born to Sandy and Jeff Smith. They were both 25 years old at the time. They had their first child when Jeff was in Vietnam and they both were 20. Their first daughter, Corie, was beautiful, blond, precocious, and intelligent—everything a first child is supposed to be. During the second pregnancy, Sandy followed all of the rules, and both parents expected another child like Corie.

Table 5-1.

Developmental Challenges for Parents of Children with Down Syndrome

Existing attitudes concerning people with handicaps developed from lifelong personal experiences (depending on amount of previous contact, family attitudes about the handicapped)

Handling the initial description and response (depending on sensitivity of professionals combined with personal experiences with people who have Down syndrome and their families)

Finding appropriate early intervention and preschool experiences (including adjustment of family schedules, transportation concerns, learning intervention techniques, meeting other families)

Getting elementary school services (including placement in the appropriate school setting))also getting piano, swimming, gymnastics, and other lessons and activities, such as scouting, for the child; getting background information and time for participating in individual education planning)

Getting appropriate middle/junior high school programming (requesting integrated setting or beginning vocational training, helping organize opportunities to develop social skills with peers, teaching and supervising bicycle and bus riding, dealing with driver license issues)

Getting appropriate secondary/vocational training (determining what will be realistic adult life goals; making preparations to work and live away from home)

Getting services to help the child when too old for public school programs (when child is slow to develop he/she continues to need adult education and relationship training)

Providing for the child's adult life and old age (including other children leaving the nest, parents becoming too old or too tired, advocacy and estate planning)

Table 5-2.

Pressures on Parents of Children with Down Syndrome

Reactions of others at all stages (including avoidance, oversympathy, projection of own concerns, response of family/friends, changes of friendship patterns, comments from acquaintances and strangers, need for someone to share the pain with)

Requests for participation in advocacy groups (including expectations of other parents and of professionals)

Finding enough time to meet this child's daily practical needs

Finding enough time for participation in lives of other children

Finding enough time for self to relax/recoup

Learning what to believe/follow from the advice of various professionals

Knowing exactly what amount of "protection" the child needs in each situation

Being able to put the diagnosis aside and know and love the child as a unique person

The pregnancy, labor, and delivery were uneventful, except that the obstetrician cautioned just prior to the birth that the baby would be quite small. But then Corie had been a small baby. The baby arrived at 12:44 a.m. The 4-pound, 9-ounce infant was breathing well, had a good Apgar reading, and had all 10 fingers and toes. The new father left the delivery room to call family members and announce the happy news.

After Jeff left, Sandy was still in the delivery room, half listening as the doctor and nurse chatted about a variety of topics. After the doctor left, the nurse came up to Sandy, patted her shoulder (the beginning of what Sandy has found to be a lifetime of "pats") and said, "I have a son 7 feet tall and still growing."

Sandy was perplexed and wondered how best to respond to the statement—"that's nice," or "that's too bad," or "he'll be great at basketball," but she smiled and said nothing at all, feigning fatigue. Sandy did not realize until later that this experienced nurse had recognized what no one else had thus far, that this tiny infant had Down syndrome.

In her own restricted way, the nurse was trying to tell Sandy that the new baby had a problem but that it would be all right. Professionalism did not allow her to say more, and the obstetrician had never delivered a child with Down syndrome before—if he suspected the diagnosis, he said nothing. Sandy did not think that there might be something wrong with her daughter. That happens to other people—not to those that take care of themselves and are good people.

In the recovery room, Sandy heard the obstetrician calling in the record of the birth. Everything was recorded as "normal," even though the baby was called premature due to her extremely small size.

That evening Jeff was there when they brought the baby to Sandy. They inspected the fingers and toes and did not notice or suspect that there was anything "different" about this baby from their first daughter. In fact, they marveled at how much their two children looked alike—not too surprising since they had the same parents!

The next morning at 9:00 a.m., Sandy was waiting for the nurse to bring Ashleigh in for her feeding. She saw through the open doors babies being shuffled up and down the hall to their mothers, but no Ashleigh. Beginning around 9:20 a.m. and frequently thereafter, Sandy rang the nurse's call button asking where her daughter was. She received a variety of answers from, "someone will be right with you, honey," to "just a moment, dear," but no explanation as to why Ashleigh was not brought to the room.

Sandy thought of reasons for the delay—a slight fever or maybe Ashleigh had been put into an incubator due to her small size—but she never considered anything serious, and certainly not "mental retardation." Finally, at about 9:45 a.m., Corie's pediatrician (who had been selected by her parents for Ashleigh also) appeared at the hospital room door. The man had been practicing for years, and he had even been Jeff's pediatrician when Jeff was a child.

The doctor was holding some papers in his hands—but no baby. Sandy's roommate was cuddling and feeding her new baby, her third. The door to the hallway was open, and the curtain between the two beds was not pulled. The doctor did not enter the room, but called Sandy's name. She had to lean forward to see him. He stood in the doorway and announced, "You have a handicapped child; she'll never be anything more than a vegetable, so my suggestion is that you sign these papers and send her away before you get attached." He continued, "Forget that you ever had her; tell people that she died; have other children; don't let her be a 'burden' on your family; she will never be a 'real' sister for your other daughter; she will be extremely delayed in everything she does." Sandy will forever remember his final words as he threw the papers on her bed, "She will never know you are her mother." By this time, the doctor's voice was loud enough for everyone to hear. Sandy's roommate started crying and clutched her newborn baby.

Once the doctor had left, Sandy rose from her bed and went into the bathroom, where she cried for what seemed an interminable amount of time. Then she walked to the window in her room and cried some more. She was shocked, horrified, enraged, and deeply grief-stricken. It was as if she were on the outside of her situation looking in—as if she had no control over what was happening.

Finally, she decided that she would go see Ashleigh and would discover for herself that the doctor was wrong. After all, Ashleigh looked much as her older sister had at birth; her parents were young, healthy, drug-free, much looking forward to this new child. Also, first and foremost, everyone knows that these things happen to other people; nothing like this had ever happened in either of their families before.

Sandy called Jeff at home, hoping that he had not left for the shopping center to buy a blanket and stuffed toy for the new baby, but there was no answer. She then took a 30-foot walk that seemed like 30 miles to the newborn nursery to prove to herself that the insensitive, harsh doctor was wrong. When she arrived at the nursery, Ashleigh was not there. Sandy knocked on the nursery window and was immediately surrounded by several well-meaning nurses patting her shoulder and trying to escort her back down the hall to her room.

Sandy asked where Ashleigh was. "We moved her to the back nursery and pulled the shades so that you wouldn't be embarrassed," Sandy was told. Sandy insisted that Ashleigh be moved to the front row of the front nursery immediately. This response was perhaps the beginning of fighting back against others' expectations of how she should feel. The nurses patted her again and quickly moved Ashleigh to the front row.

Sandy stared long and hard at her little 4-pound baby girl and could not see anything wrong with the pretty baby. She tried to disregard what the doctor had said. He was just uncaring and uninformed and had been out of medical school too long. She went back to her room, sat on her bed, and thought about the words the doctor had spoken. Although Sandy did not trust this physician, she had a constant subconscious thought that he was right. To this day, Sandy cannot tell you why she felt that way, but it was sufficient to force her into the next steps of acceptance, i.e., depression, anger, and grieving.

Sandy went to wait for Jeff at the doors of the maternity floor, and when he got off the elevator and crossed the hall, she was no longer crying. As he came through the door, he looked at her face and said, "She died, didn't she?" And then Sandy had to tell the man she loved, the father of her children, the person with whom she intended to spend the rest of her life, that his newborn daughter had a serious disability.

They sat talking for hours in the father's waiting room (having no place private to go), stopping only when an expectant or new father entered. Not only did they want, need, and deserve privacy in this most personal situation, but they were quite conscious of the joy the other families were experiencing and in no way wanted to damage that joy. Earlier that morning, when everyone on the maternity floor heard the diagnosis and prognosis for Ashleigh, there had been more than enough sharing of the pain.

What should have been a joyous time for all of the new and expectant families was dampened by the harsh intrusion of reality and vulnerability. Sandy and Jeff did not deserve their private business publicized, nor did the other families deserve to lose any of their joy and hope.

One of the labor-delivery nurses brought Sandy a 1942 textbook that had some information in it about Down syndrome, but, as might be expected, it was terribly outdated and depressed Jeff and Sandy even more. Also, they did not know anyone with a child with Down syndrome to talk to.

There was lengthy discussion about the impact this child would have on their marriage, on Corie and future children, on their career and educational goals, and on their extended family. Having gotten married at 19 and having had their first child at 20 had stopped them from finishing college—which both wanted to do. Jeff had enrolled in the local university upon his return from Vietnam and had gone to night school for 4 years before Ashleigh's birth. He had 2 more years of night school to earn a degree, then Sandy was to begin. They both had adequate jobs but wanted better; they had a nice home but wanted better, etc. Could they have any of these things if they brought Ashleigh home? Retrospectively, neither parent recalls seriously considering using the papers the doctor had left for institutionalization.

They finally decided that there were no answers and that the success of their marriage and other goals still lay with them—not with Ashleigh's diagnosis nor prognosis. Jeff left the hospital around midnight that night— neither wanting him to go; they desperately needed to be together. After she was sure that Jeff had had enough time to get home and settled, Sandy called him and could tell that he had been crying—the first time all day. He reported that he had looked up Down syndrome in a journal, which had the disability under the broad heading of *monster*.

Jeff and Sandy began to realize that the rest of their lives would be a series of peaks and valleys. Already there had been the high upon their daughter's birth and the valley upon hearing her diagnosis, climbing out of that valley when Sandy went down the hall to see the baby, slipping down again on finding her in the back nursery, etc. But with each valley, they learned to climb up faster and higher than the time before, until they reached a level where they would be able to operate on a daily basis.

Two days after Ashleigh's birth, Sandy checked out of the hospital to go home with Jeff, getting away from people who badly wanted and needed her to be brave, who did not want to see her pain, who did not know what to do for her. Ashleigh had to stay in the hospital, as she had lost weight, and Corie remained at her grandparents where she had been since Ashleigh's arrival. The house was quiet and seemed strange upon Sandy and Jeff's entrance. They walked back to the nursery and looked around at the bright, cheery room. The room was intended for a future president, an accountant, a lawyer, a physician, a waitress, or a truck driver—whatever their imagined child wanted to be. It was in this room that they bid farewell to that child, grieved her passing, and started dealing forthrightly with the child they were actually bringing home.

THE SEARCH FOR SERVICES

The next morning, Sandy and Jeff began calling service agencies to find one that could help them with their new daughter. After 12 painful conversations, in which they had to relive their daughter's diagnosis and prognosis, they finally got in touch with the appropriate service provider for newborns with disabilities such as Down syndrome. They made an appointment to visit with the person in charge of what was then called "infant stimulation." This was the beginning of a new way of life.

It was painful for Sandy and Jeff to walk through a door marked "Association for Retarded Children" and know that they were going there for *their* tiny newborn baby. It was painful when they asked the pediatrician for a prescription for an occupational/physical therapy evaluation and received a note that read, "the child cannot be helped." It was painful to see Ashleigh's first psychological evaluation reporting everything she could do in four lines and everything she could not do in four pages. And it was painful to complete each step only to find that there were always more steps to take. For the Smiths, as for other parents, there was a constant search for services that were never quite adequate.

REACTION OF OTHERS

Sandy and Jeff received a tearful phone call from the obstetrician saying how sorry he was—and pots of flowers and sympathy cards from people they did not even know. They did not know what to say to friends who were unaware of the diagnosis when they called with congratulations.

A few weeks later, some Christmas cards came addressed to Sandy, Jeff, and Corie—even from those who had been sent an announcement of Ashleigh's birth.

There were stares from people in shopping centers, and the carry-out boy in the grocery store said Ashleigh looked like a monkey. But none of these reactions were as important as the responses Jeff got when he called extended family members and close friends to tell of Ashleigh's diagnosis and prognosis. When her grandfather first saw Ashleigh, he said, "She doesn't *look* like a freak."

THE IMPORTANCE OF GRANDPARENTS

Grandparents hold their own special relationship not only to the grandchild but also to their own grown child. Grandparents also have a variety of reactions and concerns when a grandchild has Down syndrome (Table 5-3).

A study of grandparent reactions (Vadasy, Fewell, & Meyer, 1986) found that most grandparents did not suspect there was a problem until they were told, with the initial message typically coming from the parents—most often from the mother.

Grandparents handle their initial reaction largely by not telling anyone and going through much the same feelings that the parents do: sadness, shock, disbelief, depression, and anger. Ironically, many of these same feelings still remain several years later, manifesting themselves in concern

Table 5-3.

Concerns of Grandparents

Own personal reaction to the hurts and disappointments concerning the grandchild

Need to help with the grandchild to increase the child's skills

Concern for their own child's additional stress

Concern for the other grandchildren's lives and needs

Concern for the grandchild's secure future

Concern about their own ability to assist through financial, emotional, and practical support

Concern for the protection of the family tree

---

not only about the grandchild with Down syndrome but also about their own grown-up child. Parents feel it is part of their job to remove pain from their children whether that pain comes from the birth of a child with special needs or some other problem. When a grandchild with a handicap is born, grandparents find themselves unable to remove the pain.

It is important to note that the bulk of the grandparents involved in the Vadasy et al. survey felt they had been given sufficient information regarding the child's diagnosis and prognosis. The bulk of them found their own way to assist the family with the child with special needs, i.e., occasional financial support, ongoing moral support, and rather infrequent direct assistance in the home and/or with the child. Overall, grandparents of children with special needs surveyed provided more financial and caregiving support for the families with a child who is handicapped than for their other children's families without special needs.

The majority of the grandparents reported that religion helped them to understand and accept their grandchild with a handicap. Part of this acceptance is, of course, due to other family members and friends who have been helpful to the grandparents. All of the grandparents in this survey reported that they eventually confided in friends about their grandchild with special needs and overwhelmingly found them supportive.

Grandparents are concerned about the child's future in the event of the death of the parents. They try to learn more about the child's disability through conferences, talking to professionals, and discussing options with the parents. The bulk of the grandparents felt the child would/should end up living with family member if the parents could not raise the child. They saw guardianship, physical problems, and behavior issues as items to be dealt with early on.

Although most grandparents reported providing greater support for the family of the grandchild with special needs, the majority felt their relationship with that particular grandchild was not a great deal different than their relationships with their other grandchildren.

Considerable insight into grandparents was gained from the survey, including the obvious fact that these people are at a stage in their lives where they can typically offer support to families in special situations. They can fit their support to their current lifestyle, strengths, abilities, and values. In general, they are quite concerned about the future of the grandchild with special needs, including the availability of good educational programs, the financial needs associated with raising this child, and a firm plan concerning living arrangements should something happen in an untimely fashion to the parents.

The grandparents surveyed clearly feel supportive and useful to the family who has a child with special needs; in some situations they wish they could do more, but overall they are satisfied with their interactions with the family who has a child with special needs. This is important since parents of children with Down syndrome need the help, encouragement, and support of their parents and other family members and friends as they meet the daily challenge of raising the child with Down syndrome.

Parents will watch very closely the attitudes of their own parents regarding this new child—will the child be accepted as a person or as a "disabled person?" Grandparents can be primary supportive agents for the new parents particularly by *not* expecting the new parents to support them. Grandparents must allow the new parents privacy and the right to cry, to feel sorry for themselves, to grieve, and to work through their feelings by experiencing the stages of denial, anger, guilt, shock, and, finally, acceptance. None of these stages should last too long; if grandparents sense that loved ones are stuck in any one stage, they can consult the early intervention program or the local Down syndrome parent group to provide counseling for the family.

SUGGESTIONS FOR PARENTS

1. Remember that your baby is a person with hopes, dreams, rights, and dignity.

2. Understand that no one knows exactly what to tell you or how to help you.

3. Understand that some people have more or less skill in expressing empathy and feeling concern for others.

4. Ask to meet other parents of children with Down syndrome to talk about how they felt and how they now feel about their child.

5. Do not be ashamed of your feelings or of sharing them.

6. Ask persons giving you advice or information to explain where they learned the information and how much personal experience they have had with people who have Down syndrome.

7. Ask questions about anything concerning your child, even though you may think they might be trivial.

8. Refuse to accept statements such as, ''They are all like that.'' Insist that your child's skills be measured individually.

9. Insist that the professional give information to both parents together and to other family members as desired.

10. Do not allow people to counsel you except in a private, comfortable place.

11. Try to respond to the stares of the public with serenity.

12. Try to respond coolly to the curious questions of friends and passers-by.

13. Make new friends if necessary so you and your child can be comfortable.

14. Realize that you may need to deal with the sorrow of the loss of the child you had hoped to have and the shock of the diagnosis of Down syndrome.

15. Do not make the needs of the child with Down syndrome shut out the needs of other family members.

16. Remember that you are dealing with your child's life, not your life. Keep the best interests of all family members in mind.

17. Do not become discouraged with yourself as you struggle to meet all the problems and feelings and to adjust and readjust. As with anything, there will be good days and bad days. Coping with this lifelong situation is difficult.

SUGGESTIONS FOR GRANDPARENTS

1. As much as you can, treat the new child just as you would any other grandchild.

2. Remember that your job is to support the family and not the other way around; find your support somewhere else.

3. Offer to make calls to service agencies that can assist the child and family.

4. Offer to accompany the new parents on their first few visits to the service agency.

5. Offer to care for the child with Down syndrome (as well as other children in the family, without discrimination) and provide appropriate stimulation.

6. Obtain and read accurate information on the disability so that you can help the new parents to learn to answer questions, and to explain the diagnosis to others.

7. Buy the same kind and amount of gifts for the new baby as for other grandchildren.

8. Ask how the child is, but do not give extraordinary attention at a cost to the other grandchildren.

9. Help the family focus on other family members as well.

CONCLUSION: FROM A PARENT'S PERSPECTIVE

Having a child with Down syndrome is not the end of the world. It is not a tragedy for the child or the family. It does not make those it affects "victims." It does not cause a lifetime of physical and mental anguish. In fact, many families report having a special kind of joy that carries them through the bad times.

Some of this joy comes from a child saying "Mama" or walking, singing, playing, or celebrating birthdays (Michaelis, 1977). When Corie saw her sister accomplish something, she said, "*We* helped her do that," and one day explained to a friend, "We love her, so what does it matter to you?" Ashleigh herself recently interrupted the dinner conversation because she wanted to announce to her family, "I have a great life and a great family." And so, it seems, do most people who have Down syndrome.

REFERENCES

Michaelis, C.T. (1977). Merry Christmas, Jim and Happy Birthday. *The Exceptional Parent, 7*, 6–7.
Vadasy, P.F., Fewell, R.R., & Meyer, D.J. (1986). Supporting extended family members' roles: Intergenerational supports provided by grandparents of handicapped children. *Journal of the Division of Early Childhood, 10*(1), 36–44.

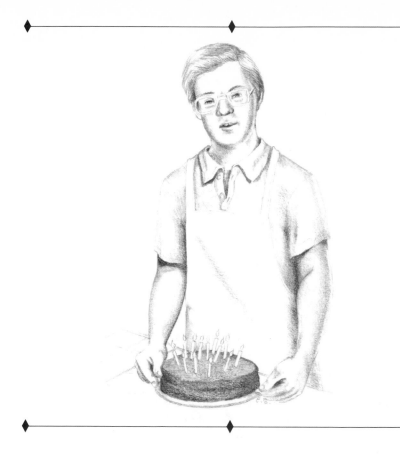

CHAPTER SIX

MY BROTHER, JIM

TRISH BOSWELL AND CAROL TINGEY

♦

Each family and each child within the family is, of course, different. Family
resources vary—not only financial resources, but also emotional resources.
Some families have many children, some only a few. Some families are
close and share their feelings with each other, some do not. Some families live in a large house, while some families share the same room. Some
families live close to grandparents, and some live in remote areas far away
from extended family and other relatives. Some live in the same house
all of their lives and others move frequently. Some families live in the city
and some in the country. None are the same. Yet each family shares feelings, and sisters and brothers have common responses that usually include
intense protectiveness toward a sister or brother with Down syndrome
along with mixed feelings of embarrassment, shame, and jealousy. Along
with these feelings almost always comes the expectation of helping.

The following is the good and bad story of one sister growing up with
a brother who has Down syndrome.

MY PRESCHOOL YEARS

I don't really remember ever suddenly discovering that Jim was "different"; to me he was just another brother. Brothers are my specialty. I
have four of them, all born before me. Jim is 4 years older than I am, and
there is a brother in between us and two older than Jim. In those early
years, we were all more concerned with ourselves than getting to know
one another, but I noticed and remembered some things. For example,
one of my grandmothers would gladly babysit all of us, except Jim. He
was driven to another town for our other, willing grandmother to tend.
Jim also went to school in a little tiny bus while my two oldest brothers
walked to school.

Of course, as time went on it became more evident that Jim was different. He used to wander off. I remember driving around in our car with
my mother frantically looking for him. By this time, we had moved to a
new city, and I was surprised by the neighbors' reactions to Jim. I guess
I just accepted him. How could I not? After all, he was as much my brother
as Dick, Blaine, or Neil were. He already had a place in my family before
I arrived. I could understand him and put up with him, even though he
wasn't always pleasant. He was like an overgrown 2-year-old. He was
immature but strong. He'd push me and my youngest brother down and
take our toys. I remember very well one day he pushed me down the stairs
several times and just laughed at me and threw something on top of me
if I didn't move.

All of this didn't really seem to be unusual. Even Jim's funny faces
and noises only amused me. Sometimes outsiders took offense to Jim.

I remember one upset neighbor lady yelling something like, "Keep *him* away from my children!" All he had done was thrown dirt clods at them. (They probably deserved it!)

Fortunately, not all neighbors were like that. One family in particular liked Jim. They made him feel so at home that he often went into their home unannounced. Over 20 years later, they still ask, "How's Jimmy?"

Soon my friends grew to be very important to me. I enjoyed having them over, and in a way Jim did too, although he chose strange ways to show it. He'd sneak up and knock my girlfriend's head and mine together. He even pushed Cindy down the back stairs. She wouldn't come over for awhile, and I couldn't blame her.

My mom was a Cub Scout den mother for at least a hundred years. I attended enough Cub Scout meetings to be almost an honorary cub (except I never got my own pinewood derby car). I know now that she didn't do it for fun. She did it for my brothers, mostly Jim. He was learning more sociably acceptable behaviors all the time. He still made occasional blunders like squeezing my kitty too tight and putting his finger through a soft turtle shell (may they rest in peace), but at least my friends would come over (we'd shut my door).

MY ELEMENTARY YEARS

I learned that Jim's handicap was something called *Down syndrome*. Those were words I didn't understand. I was more affected by the terms, *Mongolism* and *Mongoloid*. They sounded disgusting but were unfortunately better known at the time. I was upset by the way Jim looked. We were constantly reminding him to keep his mouth closed with his tongue in it. He was also very slow. He took a long time in the bathroom and a long time to get ready to go places. He would sometimes refuse to go somewhere if he didn't have enough time to get himself mentally ready. He also had strange idiosyncrasies like tapping his fingers against his lips and bouncing his head on his pillow before going to sleep at night. Despite these oddities, I loved Jim and felt like I should take care of him.

In elementary school, I began to fill an older sister role. I became very protective toward Jim. I taught Jim to refer to me as his favorite (not only) sister (bless his heart, he still says that). I called him my "big, little brother." When Mom left us alone, we'd argue who was in charge—sometimes I let Jim believe it was him.

One morning as I walked Jim to his bus stop (it was my job), a most memorial incident happened. A boy in my class from school who lived near the bus stop saw us and came out. He started throwing rocks at Jim and yelled to me, "You're retarded because your brother is." He said it several times, almost chanting it. I can still hear it now. I got Jim safely on the bus and went home. I remember many kids being called "retarded," but this was different—it hit home. I remember that it hurt for a long time; in fact, I'm not sure I'm over it now.

I used to love to play school. My grandmother, who was a teacher, gave me some old teachers' books, and I became the teacher. Jim was my favorite student. We worked with the old basal readers for a while, then I'd ring a bell for recess and we'd stop for awhile and start again later. I'd had half the little neighbor kids in school also. Jim and I both love kids. He seems to have patience with them, and they cautiously warmed up to him.

About that time, Neil (our brother in between) was also growing up and deciding what to do about Jim. Jim loved sports (our older brother, Blaine, was a high school basketball player, and Jim loved following his every game). Neil was in Little League baseball and a pretty good player. The whole family went to most of the games. Jim got excited when Neil made a good play. He'd cheer him on, usually by standing up, yelling, and almost dancing. If Neil hit a home run, Jim got excited and went to home plate to hug and congratulate Neil. This embarrassed Neil, and he told mother to grab Jim if he made a home run so Jim would not go to home plate. We found out later that Neil had told a teammate that Jim was adopted. Somehow, that made Neil feel better.

I guess we all wondered why Jim had come to our family. Blaine had asked, "Why him and not me?" I remember hearing that Jim had been tested and that there was no hereditary reason that he ended up the way he was—it was an accident. I felt torn between wanting to protect him and being embarrassed about him.

This frustrating feeling of liking Jim but not liking Jim came up at odd times. One time when I was mad at Jim, I stomped on his foot with my tap shoes as hard as I could. I felt guilty for years because that night he got rheumatic fever in that ankle and I thought that I had caused him to get it (which wasn't possible). I would get mad at myself for getting mad at him. He did plenty of things to get mad at, too. He would take my things. He loved to take my Barbie dolls. I would find them under his bed without their clothes on. I think he was discovering what an idealistic body Barbie had, but I was upset because they were my favorite toys and I was very careful with them. Santa even brought Jim a Ken doll, but that obviously didn't solve the problem!

Jim would talk to himself or think out loud. I guess we all talk to ourselves or think out loud, but Jim would answer himself as well. He'd say things such as, "I need to go to the bathroom...yah, I need to go to the bathroom." If he was busy in his bedroom, we could usually tell exactly what he was doing by the play-by-play commentary. He also used to do whole baseball games in which he would be the pitcher, the batter, the umpire, the crowd, and both teams' fans. If we bothered him during these games he would scold us, even for calling him to dinner. After the games he would come inside (when there was good weather, the games were held outside) and announce who was the winner. Sometimes when he didn't tell us, we'd ask; those were usually the days that his favorite team had lost.

Going to one of Jim's school carnivals or programs was always an experience. We other kids would sometimes come home imitating the chorus's off-key singing and discussing some of Jim's classmates. I didn't really mind going because we rarely would see any of the people that lived in our neighborhood or went to our school. And the people that were there knew what it was like to have a retarded person in their family— they understood. Besides, it was a night to honor Jim. As busy as the rest of us were going to practices and dancing lessons and games and recitals, Jim deserved a few nights of his own.

Jim had some friends from school who would come over to the house every once in a while. Jim would take a minute to say hi; then he would do his own thing and not really interact any more. Some of his friends would do the same, and others would visit with the rest of us. We began to label Jim's friends as "look-alikes" (people with Down syndrome) and "not look-alikes." Jim understood and talked about his school friends the same way. He was never wrong.

Every summer Jim went to camp for 2 weeks. He looked forward to it all year. One of his favorite buddies was Bobby (who was a look-alike). They would greet each other at the bus with great hugs (it's true that people with Down syndrome are affectionate). I remember feeling glad that he had somewhere fun to go and that *we* could have a break from him. He came home after camp the first year with 13 days worth of clean clothes and wearing the same outfit he had worn when left. The poor counselor apologized, but no need, we understood. Even after soaking and washing, Mom couldn't get that outfit clean. I think she just threw the whole mess away.

Jim has had numerous girlfriends. The first was the famed Barbara. She was not a look-alike but evidently that was not required by Jim. The two were on the phone hours almost daily. They never really talked, just made noises to each other. Neil and I more than once were scolded by an angry brother in love because we liked to listen on another phone and imitate the sounds and add a few kissy sounds. Who's to say that was not just ordinary sibling rivalry? We liked teasing him just as much as we liked teasing each other.

As we all grew taller every year, Jim began to associate height with age. Therefore, he thought, if someone is older, they are also taller. I think he knew Neil and I had passed him up mentally, and he wanted to make sure we didn't forget he was really older. He'd still say his height is 5'8" (just taller than me) when he is really only 5'6". He will, however, let little brother Neil be over 6 feet tall. Dick and Blaine are also taller than Jim, but that is okay with Jim because they are older.

Numbers have always been Jim's thing. He memorizes sports statistics. He knows baseball players' batting averages, basketball players' average points per game, and football players' height and weight. He can recite these at any time. He also knows birthdays or someone's exact age if he heard it once.

Sometimes when friends would come over, I would encourage Jim to display his knowledge to show that he had talents too. This probably did two things; it made Jim aware of what he could share with people, and it helped me to be able to think of him of someone special rather than someone who couldn't do anything worthwhile.

I was then (and I still am) very selective about who I tell I have a retarded brother. When asked about my family, I would say that I had four older brothers. I might have mentioned that three of them were in high school instead of saying that Jim went to a special school. Other times I would wait to get to know someone to see if I could trust him or her before I said anything. I would rarely tell someone I just met. I guess I learned at a young age that some people don't understand or are quick to tease.

JUNIOR HIGH YEARS

Going into seventh grade is a dramatic experience for most 12-year-olds. I think it was the end of my belief that everyone lives happily ever after. Beside changing schools that year, I learned or maybe just realized that growing up was hard. I guess I also realized that Jim wasn't going to grow up with me and that might be difficult for both of us.

Our family went through some drastic changes that year. My older two brothers went away to college, and my parents divorced. So it was Mom, Jim, Neil, and me. It was a time of adjustments. I tried to sort out the reasons for my parents' divorce, wondering if it was something I did. I worried that maybe Jim was the cause. One of my older brothers was angry with my mom and often voiced this on weekend visits. It was a time of unrest in our household. Jim, Neil, and I were supposed to spend every other weekend with our dad.

I went through periods when I felt I had two things to hide: Jim and the *divorce*. Visitation was really bad. I couldn't go to parties or felt I couldn't go because it was the weekend with Dad. I missed my mom and didn't want her to be alone. My dad lived in a small condominium, and I didn't feel like I had the privacy that a girl my age needed. I was embarrassed to tell any of my friends. I guess divorce wasn't as well accepted then as it seems to be now.

I guess this is when I began to feel that I was a second mother to Jim. My dad didn't take care of Jim the way my mom did, so on those weekends I took care of him. I made sure his bags were packed and that he had everything he needed and wanted. I would bring along his Matchbox cars, which he still enjoyed (even though he was 16). I would make sure that he took his bath and changed his clothes. I even shaved his face where he missed spots. I interpreted things that he said that others could not understand. If my dad had a question about Jim he'd ask me. I was becoming the expert on Jim away from home.

I also worried a lot about my life at that time. I was curious about and interested in boys like my girlfriends were and spent hours talking with them. I wondered about the changes in my body and how to wear my hair. I had to get my ears pierced because my best friend did. I wondered if I should wear makeup and which kind looked better. I giggled and I cried. My every-other-weekend role was very responsible and grown-up and somehow sandwiched into these unsure times.

After my eighth-grade year, my mom packed us up and we moved to another state. This seemed like a good way to escape the weekends with my dad and I was glad of that, but this also took us away from the neighbors who knew us; even if they didn't like Jim (which most of them did) they already knew him and we didn't have to do any explaining. It was hard for me to leave my friends as I'm sure it was for Neil (in fact, he very much wanted to stay, and I was afraid he might). I guess I shared the worries with my mom on how Jim would take the change, but I think he was ready to go before we were. One day a neighbor called and Jim answered the phone. When she asked for Mom, Jim announced, "We moved to Iowa," and then hung up. He had been thinking about it and he was ready.

We sat down after that first day of new schools to discuss how it had gone. Neil and I had both arranged to try out for the basketball teams. I compared my last band teacher with my new one. Then we asked Jim how his day had gone. We asked about the bus and if there were any look-alikes on it. There were some. He also mentioned a student he described as being "sort of brown" (he had never seen a black person before). All and all, things were going to be just fine. Some things never change—Jim still took a long time in the bathroom and was slow getting ready to go places.

Soon after we moved, there we met a young family that had just had a child. Their child also had Down syndrome. We became good friends with them. They watched Jim very carefully, wondering if their new baby would someday be like the big 18-year-old boy. They also decided that maybe they could have more babies because, of course, Neil and I had come after Jim. I loved to hold their baby, and I wondered if Jim was just as cute and helpless as Tommy was at that point.

Neil made the basketball team. He remembered the Little League games with Jim and decided in this new chance for fame Jim was not to be involved. Jim had to stay home. I must admit I wasn't allowed to go either, but I didn't want to. I felt bad for Jim, who would never play on a high school team and who loved to follow the sports—especially if a beloved brother was involved. Jim would wait at the door for my mother (the only one allowed to go) to return with a printed program so he could review with the program what he had heard on the radio. I was angry at Neil, and I didn't understand all the feeling that he may have had.

Jim could take care of things that didn't appeal to him in his life. The bus driver was supposed to pick up his riders in front of their houses, but Jim didn't like that. He would simply wait at the corner and soon that was his stop. He also decided to play hooky every once in a while. Some mornings he would put the sign in the window that signaled the bus to go on without him.

Jim definitely has a will of his own as I found out on our first adventure being travel buddies. The first summer after we moved we went back for a month of visitation with our dad. Neil had flown out earlier, so it was just Jim and me on our very first plane ride. Jim found the first leg of our journey very interesting and talked aloud to himself about the things he saw. I was slightly embarrassed and kept shushing him. I felt relieved after we successfully changed planes in Denver. I was nervous about doing something I had never done before and also about being totally responsible for my big, talk-to-himself, slow, clumsy, retarded brother. On the second plane they served us a snack. Jim sure loves food. I don't know why they served us wine. I was definitely underage, and Jim didn't act or look his age. I just wasn't going to drink mine, and I assumed Jim would do the same, but I guess suggestive advertising had gotten to him. I begged him not to drink and he would just smile. The other passengers were noticing my plight; I pleaded with him. He opened his one serving bottle and drank the whole thing. Snickers were coming from the seats around us. Jim had won.

During our visit with dad, I kept Jim very near me. I sensed that if I kept Jim out of the way things would be better. My dad had gotten remarried that summer. There was a stepmother and her children to get to know. I don't think anyone was comfortable. Jim and I were both glad to go home. Fortunately they didn't serve wine on the return flight.

I think that next year Neil and I felt more comfortable in our school setting. We both started dating. Neil would go out with girls from school and usually never brought them home. I have a feeling that he never mentioned Jim to them. He was still very uncomfortable. I think he liked

Jim but was never sure what people would think of him if they knew. I, on the other hand, started by dating someone who was a friend of the family and already acquainted with Jim.

That spring my mom was very ill. I took care of our household. I visited her in the hospital. I even figured her college students' grades for the term. I was really frightened at the time. I knew if I lost her I would miss her very much and I would be Jim's only mother instead of his second mother. Fortunately, she recovered and took care of us again, but I think that incident made me realize that Jim was going to be my responsibility some day. I knew that it wasn't something that I had a choice about. I may have only been 16 on the outside, but inside I was an ageless adult with responsibilities.

One day about that time I saw something that changed my feelings about being seen with Jim in public. I was in a shopping mall when I saw two girls walking down the mall. I noticed that one of them was leading the other one, who was carrying a white cane and was blind. I decided as they came closer that they were sisters. The sister that was leading walked with upright posture and held her head high. I realized that she knew people like me were looking at her and her sister but was proud, not embarrassed. I decided that I could do that, too. From then on I was proud of what Jim could accomplish instead of embarrassed by his handicaps. It's funny—after that Jim's physical characteristics became "his" instead of those of a person with Down syndrome. I admit that are were times that I don't feel that way, but most of the time I do.

HIGH SCHOOL

Just before my junior year in high school, we moved again. This time I took it as a challenge. I looked at it as a contest to see how many friends I could make that would sign my yearbook at the end of the year. Jim also seemed quite adaptable to new situations by then, too. Besides, he had expressed that he wanted to work instead of doing crafts like his last school did. The school he entered was called a high school and he liked that.

Jim and I still occasionally argued over who was oldest or in charge. After I got my driver's license, I liked to rub it in. Jim had an earlier experience that although minor had convinced him that he did not want to drive. I would say to him, "Ha, ha, I can drive and you can't!" Sometimes he would push me or tell me to shut up. He could push me real hard; he is very strong. I knew my behavior was mean, and I felt bad that I said those things and hurt his feelings, but I still did it every once in a while.

Food was getting to be a problem. Jim just ate everything! He would even take money from our wallets or use his own to buy food at the local grocery store. Finally, we decided to do something drastic. We bought chains and locks and locked up the cupboards and the refrigerator. My friends would comment about it being strange, but it became a way of life for us.

I could tell when Jim didn't like my friends. A couple of girls came over one day and they were a bit snotty. I don't think they even said hello to Jim, and he evidently didn't like that. When the girls went to leave, we could not find their purses, which we had left on the couch. I questioned Jim. He had a funny look on his face. We finally found the purses in the laundry basket in the basement. The girls may never understand, but Jim had expressed his feelings effectively.

I guess I should have realized that other people did not enjoy, understand, or accept Jim the way I did. My steady boyfriend my senior year asked me to go to a university basketball game. Since I had to work, I suggested that maybe he could take Jim with his extra ticket. He took Jim, and I didn't hear until months after we broke up how embarrassed he was. He said Jim would stand up and yell for the team and wouldn't sit down when asked (maybe *he* could empathize with Neil). I am still glad that Jim had a good time, and I thought it was sweet that my boyfriend would do that for me (who knows, though, maybe that's why he broke up with me).

That year I also had it out with my dad. Blaine got married during spring break. My dad said he had only enough money to fly me out to the wedding, not Jim, too. (By this time, Neil had graduated from high school and was going to college close to where Dad lived). It had been a bad 3 months for Jim. The school only let Jim go until he turned 21 in December, and there were waiting lists for sheltered workshops. I, on the other hand, was having the time of my life in my senior year. The contrast bothered me, and I thought Jim deserved to go. I ended up going alone. When I got there I observed several times when my dad forgot that Jim was not there or didn't think of him as his son. He made the comment that he was glad that he had *all* his children with him. I started to cry, and the thought occurred to me that perhaps my Dad didn't just love his kids because they were his. Maybe he had invited me because I looked all right and wouldn't embarrass him. I didn't want to believe this. Unfortunately, I would have many more reminders of my father's lack of interest in Jim in the future.

Jim and I shared graduation. Although Jim was through in December, they let him come back to graduation in June. It could have ended up being another I'm-older-than-you problem, but, fortunately, Jim's graduation was the day before mine. Whew! In the newspaper on the page that printed the names of the graduates, my mom had two of us! Our diplomas were identical. Does that mean he had learned the same skills as I did? I didn't know it then, but the diplomas would lead Jim with me to college!

COLLEGE

I had decided to attend a university back in the state where I went to elementary school. It was in the same town in which my grandparents lived. It was decided that I would live in an apartment in their house to save money. Later it was decided that Jim would come with me. He was still on the waiting lists for adult services but there were 600 names ahead of his. Since my grandma was involved in special education (she went back to school after Jim was born to become a special education teacher), she could get him in her local sheltered workshop. So off to college *we* went.

We had only enough money for us to go by bus. It was a 4-day journey across the country. My mom and some friends came to the bus stop to wave us on. As we pulled out, Jim began his personal conversations (out loud). Then he started tapping his lip with his fingers. I began to look around to see if anyone was noticing when I realized everyone else had strange habits as well. I then felt grateful that I had Jim to protect me from them. I went with that thought until we reached Omaha at 3:00 A.M., then I suggested to Jim that he change his underclothes during the scheduled 30-minute stop. He went in the restroom and 25 minutes later he came out. During those 25 minutes I debated many things in my mind that might have happened to Jim to take him so long. Somebody had knifed him. He fell asleep. He was having difficulty moving at that hour. I walked back and forth in front of the men's room that whole time. People were probably wondering about me. Just when I was about to go in, out came Jim with a smile on his face, ready to go. I had forgotten how slow he is!

When we finally arrived, it was on the eve of Neil's departure to Texas. He was going to work there for a while. Excited that we could see him before he left, I was disappointed to hear that Neil had called and asked that Jim not be at the airport the next day. Well, after my 4-day experience, I was not about to have Jim left out of anything—so I brought him along. At the airport I realized Neil's dilemma. There was his girlfriend, who had promised to wait for Neil to come back and marry her. Evidently she had not been told that Jim existed—let alone that he was Neil's brother. I think Neil was the one who should have been left home!

Grandma was all excited to have us come, but Grandpa took some convincing. Grandma and I tried to make it as comfortable as possible. Things were going pretty well by Christmas when my mom came out to visit. I liked it when she visited—it gave me relief from being responsible for Jim. One morning just after the holidays Grandpa couldn't find his false teeth, which he kept in a cup on top of the john. When questioned, Jim explained that he had wanted to use the glass and had poured the water into the john while the john was flushing. The teeth were gone. Well, Grandma, Mom, and I braced ourselves to tell Grandpa, knowing how apprehensive he had been earlier about Jim. We were terrifically relieved when Grandpa laughed and laughed and said he needed some new teeth anyway. Jim had won his heart.

I was missing some of the roommate experience of going to college, so I asked if one of my childhood friends could come and live with us. My grandparents' house had been divided into apartments so my roommate and I would have our own kitchen. This kitchen was located next to Jim's room. After a few trusting nights I went and bought locks and chains to lock the refrigerator and cupboards. We also made sure that Jim reimbursed us with money earned at the workshop whenever he raided our cupboards.

A little gold-colored car was mine if I drove Jim everywhere he needed to go and also took Grandma on her errands. It sounded like a pretty good deal, only there were definitely strings attached. I got the privilege of driving the Special Olympic car pool. Every young adult should have the experience of having a retarded man wetting his pants in the back seat of the car only to help him out to throw up in the gutter and look up to see his speechless, humiliated, and embarrassed mother standing there.

About a year and a half after we came, Jim was able to get into a group home situation. The first one was with a young family and two other retarded men that Jim affectionately called *homemates*. To help out with things, I offered to babysit with the group home parent's own baby, and I also made sure Jim had a ride to Grandma's house and back on Friday evenings (which at times interfered with dating).

The first family tried but had their trials. A few things they did upset me. They had Jim in a converted garage that had no other way to get to the bathroom than to go outside and in the front door. During the winter that was cruel, as it was just too cold. Also, one of the other men would lock Jim out of the house. Well, everyone got upset when they realized Jim was simply going to the bathroom in his metal waste basket. I also felt that Jim, who loves food, was not getting enough. You could see his ribs. My mom, grandma, and I discussed these things with the social worker assigned to Jim. She wasn't really much help. By the looks of her office, she was more interested in pizza (she had a menu pinned up for every parlor in town).

The next family Jim was placed with seemed to be determined to do better. Jim got more food and the bathroom was closer (although I found out he was throwing away any underwear that got dirty—after buying more, I told him to stop). On one Friday night visit, I discovered some bruises on Jim's neck. I asked Jim about it but got a confused answer. So I asked the family. They told me some story about some man who gave Jim a lift and beat him. It sounded fishy, so I asked one of the other retarded man who had lived there and was more verbal than Jim. He said that the father of the family often came home after a bad day and hit everyone and often left bruises. I went to state my case to the social worker, and she said that if Jim moved he would lose his spot and not be able to live in a group home anymore. With my grandparents getting older I knew Jim needed this home. When I started to cry the social worker told me that nobody cares as much as the family does. Fortunately, the group home parents decided not to do it anymore, and we got acquainted with new ones.

By this time, I had also moved out of my grandparents' house. One day I got a call from the family that Jim lived with telling me that he had been put in the hospital. No one seemed to know what was wrong. I went to the hospital and was met by a nervous neurologist who had never worked with a person who had Down syndrome. They thought Jim had a seizure. This nervous doctor pulled me out in the hall to ask me, a "college kid," what was wrong. I knew that whenever Jim was sick he was incoherent, so maybe he didn't have a seizure and was just saying how he felt. When the doctor and I walked back into the room I discovered that Jim had urinated in the cover that goes over his dinner. The doctor didn't know what to think. I guess Jim was just too weak to get up!

We found out that Jim had rheumatic fever for the third time. At this time I needed some moral support, and since my father only lived an hour away I asked him to come up. During my dad's visit he saw how upset I was and in his effort to console me he said, "Don't worry or get attached to Jim, he'll just die soon anyway." I was so shocked, because I would worry more and be more concerned if I did know he was going to die—I love him and would want every last minute with him. Again I was faced with the fact that my dad never accepted Jim and even believed old stories that suggested that people with Down syndrome die young. At that time Jim was 25 years old. He recovered completely. I learned never to count on my dad for moral support. I also knew that the divorce was necessary.

On campus I was known as "Miss Information," due to my job at the information desk. It was a fun job. It allowed me to be where the action was. One night the action was a state Special Olympics dance. I could see the dance floor from my desk. The athletes were hopping and bopping to many different beats, some even to the beat of the music. Jim was there with his girlfriend at the time. Her name was Sherry and she called me "Jim's sister." While I was enjoying this scene I recognized an old friend. It was Bobby from the going-to-camp days. I somehow got his attention and asked him if he remembered Jim. He did. I pointed Jim out on the dance floor and told Bob to go say hi. I watched the now bald-headed man walk toward Jim. They gave each other a great big bear hug and then turned and walked in opposite directions. I just bawled...they remembered each other but they were unable to communicate what they were doing now. Things are different for Jim and Bob than for me. I wondered how many things they really miss—or am I the one missing things?

In my college, there was someone in my English class that I knew from elementary school. I tried to sit on the opposite side of the room from him—I hoped he didn't recognize me. Then one day we ended up having to work in a small group together for just a few minutes. He said hello, but I ignored him. I couldn't say hello to him—he was the one who had called me and Jim retarded many years earlier, and I would never forgive him. He probably doesn't even remember saying it. Some wounds are deep. I didn't even give him a chance to tell me what he was doing now.

One of my boyfriends really liked Jim. Bart would take Jim to Grandma's on Fridays if I was working. He would invite Jim to go out with us. I remember one pizza and a movie that was fun except that I noticed half the pizza was still in Jim's fingernails. They were longer than mine, so I took a minute and cut them. As fate goes, Bart wasn't the one for me. The night I broke up with Bart he told me that I shouldn't break up with him because I would never find anyone who would like Jim as well as he did. I knew as well as Bart that Jim would be a factor in deciding whom I would marry, but I decided to take the chance on someone else having a good relationship with Jim.

The year before I graduated from Utah State University, my mom came to teach there. This was a terrific thing to happen. I would not be solely responsible for Jim anymore. For 4 years I had this duty. If people didn't know what to get Jim for Christmas or his birthday they would ask me. If Jim was invited to a family party, it was my duty to get him there and take care of him. Now I could really get down to graduating and I could move out of town if I wanted to.

I graduated in elementary education in June of 1984. I had a job already lined up in the state's capital city. I was surprised to hear from several family members and close friends how they were glad that I didn't go into special education because of Jim. They thought I had done my duty and so did I. I think some people thought I might feel like I should be helping Jim more. I guess I never thought I'd have enough patience for that, or maybe I felt overqualified.

I met Brent my last quarter at Utah State University. We dated for 2 years before we were engaged. He was the man I wanted, but Bart had been right. Brent wasn't as enthusiastic about Jim as he was. It took Brent a while before he felt comfortable around Jim. Brent and I discussed the possibilities of Jim being our responsibility some day. It wasn't an easy thing to accept. As time went on, things worked out. I asked Brent if he minded having a person with Down syndrome collecting the gifts at our wedding. Brent thought for a while and then said that no, he didn't want to go out and recruit a person with Down syndrome to gather gifts at our wedding, but if Jim was available he'd like him to.

When I told Jim that I was going to get married, he said, "Oh, to Bart," even though that had been years before. I was worried about Brent and

Jim's relationship until one day Jim looked up at Brent and said, "Hello, brother-in-law."

Jim wore diapers at the same time I did, he graduated from high school at the same time I did, and he came to college with me. I think he was jealous the day I got married. He came home and, before my mother noticed, took my wedding announcement and threw it away. He told my mom the wedding was over and he wanted to go to work the next day. I don't know if Jim will ever get the chance to get married. I know he'd like to.

Jim is doing well at the workshop. He is washing dishes at the university's cafeteria. I don't think these are permanent things. I'd like to see him working out in the real world; he's a good worker and he should be challenged more. I'm happy when he's happy. I know that some day he might be my responsibility again, and I am willing to do whatever it takes, but right now I am enjoying taking care of my husband and myself.

PART 3
EARLY DEVELOPMENT

As infants with Down syndrome develop, more than just their physical appearance sets them apart from other children. There are differences in development, which in the early years are particularly apparent in the areas of motor and language skills. These early skills are extremely important to overall development. Through them children discover themselves and their surroundings, and they learn how to interact verbally and nonverbally with people and things in their environment. Because of the impact early development has on later learning, early intervention can be crucial to later physical and cognitive development of children with Down syndrome.

Two specific aspects of early development, covered in Chapters 7 and 8 respectively, are gross motor and speech and language development. Motor development progresses from gross movements to achievement of fine motor control. The attainment of self-care, social, recreational, and work skills depends on the ability to effectively use hands, arms, legs, and other body parts. It is important to note that there are enormous variations in the abilities of all children, and that no child has every problem. The problems discussed are typical physical development problems encountered by children with Down syndrome. For each child specific problems must be identified by an evaluation by an experienced therapist.

People with Down syndrome have difficulty with language and speech. They have difficulty with understanding words, with the combination of words, and in producing the sounds of words. Because of this difficulty, people with Down syndrome can experience problems in understanding and making themselves understood, and may as a result become isolated, especially from those who do not know them well. One of the most intimate of all human needs is that of being with people with whom one can share thoughts and feelings. Understanding the language and speech difficulties of people with

Down syndrome will help others to organize communication settings that facilitate optimal speech and language development and production. Language is discussed in Chapter 8.

The final chapter in this section, Chapter 9, covers the evolution of early intervention programs. Not only the child, but the entire family, receives aid from early services. It is stressed that families and service providers must work together to develop the most effective ways of meeting the needs of all members of the family, including, of course, the child with Down syndrome.

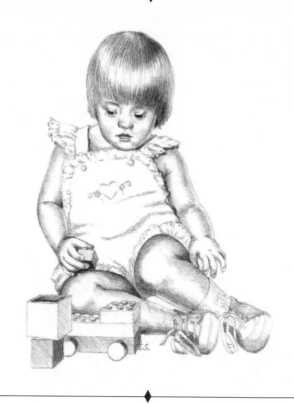

CHAPTER SEVEN

GROSS MOTOR DEVELOPMENT IN YOUNG CHILDREN WITH DOWN SYNDROME

CAROL NIMAN-REED AND
DIXIE H. SLEIGHT

This chapter focuses on the gross motor development of the infant and young child with Down syndrome. The general characteristics of gross motor performance as well as specific gross motor patterns of movement are described. In addition, activities are included for modifying and enhancing motor skills. This information is organized in developmental stages, beginning with infancy and progressing through early childhood.

The reader should remember that there is enormous variance in children's abilities and that the following descriptions of motor behavior are a compilation of observations of many children with Down syndrome. Consequently, only portions of the information included will be applicable to an individual child.

GENERAL CHARACTERISTICS

The development of gross motor skills concerns most parents of children with Down syndrome because of the child's slower achievement of motor milestones. This delay in development is less noticeable in infancy but becomes more apparent as the child gets older. As motor milestones such as walking and running are accomplished, the child with Down syndrome may not appear as coordinated or agile as other children.

The sequencing of gross motor milestones in children with Down syndrome often varies from the typical pattern of development. The most common variation is the tendency to omit creeping on hands and knees and to substitute alternate locomotion patterns including crawling on the stomach, rolling, or ''walking'' by scooting on the hips while sitting. Not only are some patterns omitted, but the child with Down syndrome spends a greater than usual amount of time in certain preferred positions, the most common being back-lying and sitting.

The child with Down syndrome prefers movement patterns that require a minimal expenditure of energy. This is a reflection of the effort required rather than a predisposition to be lazy. Often, movement is downward with gravity rather than upward against gravity. The body is frequently fully supported on a surface as in rolling or crawling on the stomach. During floor play, the child with Down syndrome is content to remain in one position for long periods of time rather than expending the energy required to change positions.

DEFICITS INFLUENCING MOTOR SKILLS

Deficits that directly influence gross motor development in children with Down syndrome are structural, sensory, and neuromotor. *Structure* refers to the physical construction of the body, while *sensory* refers to the perception of touch, balance, and vision. *Neuromotor* relates to the central nervous system's influence on movement. (Note: Many of the terms used in this discussion are explained in the glossary found on page 117.)

Structure

Three structural defects that affect gross motor skills are (1) shortened bones throughout the body, (2) instability of the vertebra of the neck (atlantoaxial instability), and (3) heart defects. The shortened bones, especially the long bones of the arms and legs, influence the child's ability to perform certain developmental tasks, such as propping on the arms in sitting and in climbing stairs.

Atlantoaxial instability is a malalignment of the first two vertebra of the neck. This is present in approximately 20 percent of all individuals with Down syndrome, and the amount of instability varies between children. When present, there is danger of damage to the spinal cord if the neck is excessively bent forward or backward with pressure (see Chapter 3). Children who have not been screened by x-ray or who have a positive x-ray should not participate in gymnastics, diving, or even doing somersaults.

The presence of a heart defect may also have significant bearing on the function of the child with Down syndrome. Children with cardiac problems have decreased endurance and are frequently irritable. They will often sleep on their stomach but resist being in prone when awake and active. They may prefer rolling as a mobility pattern and vigorously resist crawling on the stomach or on all fours. The child with a heart defect should be closely monitored during gross motor tasks, and his or her program should be consistent with the recommendation of the cardiologist.

Sensory Systems

Sensory systems that influence movement include those that monitor touch, the force and direction of movement, and balance as well as vision. *Tactile* refers to the ability to feel where and with what the body has been touched. *Proprioception* concerns the relationship of body parts to one another and provides information about the force, speed, and direction of movement. The *vestibular system* monitors the center of gravity and directs motor responses that maintain and restore balance. *Vision* serves to direct movement and provides information concerning the relation of the body to other objects. Sensory information is integrated by the brain to provide a person with a precise picture of his or her body as it moves about in the environment.

For example, when a child throws a bean bag at a target, the proprioceptive system monitors the force and direction of the movement of the arm. The tactile system focuses on the moment when the hand releases the bag, and the vestibular system controls balance during the weight shift required for throwing. Finally, the visual system provides feedback as to the success of the effort.

Many children with Down syndrome over- or underrespond to sensory input. Both underresponsiveness and overresponsiveness interfere with the ability to learn. With underresponsiveness, the awareness of input is so diminished that the child is not adequately aroused and focused for learning. Alternately, the hyperresponsive child interprets input as unpleasant or uncomfortable and avoids participating in activities. In both cases, learning through the senses is impaired.

Tactile

In the infant with Down syndrome, hyporesponsiveness to touch is characterized by decreased awareness and attention to input from the sensation of touch. The child may not put his or her hand or objects in the mouth for exploration. Toys and surfaces are only briefly touched and handled. As the child matures, the ability to use the tactile system for discrimination and manipulation of objects does not become precise.

The child who is hyperresponsive to touch is referred to as tactually defensive. This child may resist handling things that are wet or slick and may avoid activities that most children enjoy. Frequently, such children cry and pull away. Many common experiences such as walking barefoot in grass, washing hands under a running faucet, or playing in the sand may be uncomfortable for children who are hyperresponsive to touch, and they may avoid doing them.

Proprioception

Hyporesponsiveness to proprioceptive input is a decreased ability to feel the position of the body as well as the force of the body's movement. In children with Down syndrome, this is especially apparent in the legs and feet. Some children do not use their legs and feet to help them move when crawling on the stomach or to assist in balance when sitting in a chair. There is a lack of awareness of the position of the feet when starting to walk and climb. Children may use the same amount of force for all tasks rather than making modifications relative to the activity. For example, they tend to throw a ball with equal force no matter what the distance to the target.

Some children with Down syndrome avoid weight bearing on the arms and legs. Children may resist weight bearing on their knees when placed in a hands and knees or four-point position. When standing is attempted, they may refuse to support their body weight on their feet and may pull their legs up and off the floor. These behaviors are referred to as *proprioceptive hyperresponsiveness*.

Vestibular

Balance reactions of children with Down syndrome may lack the quickness necessary to meet the demands of a wide range of gross motor activities. Often, the feet may be wider apart than usual during walking, providing a more secure base of support. If they fall, movement of the arms to break the fall and protect the body may not be completely present. The arms may not fully extend or the response may not be present in all directions (forward, sideways, backwards). When children with Down syndrome fall, they often hyperextend their necks backwards, arch their backs, and roll forward on their stomachs rather than extending their arms to catch themselves.

Children who have excessive fear of heights and unstable or moving surfaces have gravitational insecurity. These children may resist swings, slides, stairs, and ramps or insist on keeping their feet on the ground. Children who exhibit gravitational insecurity may be unwilling to climb, may verbalize fear of falling, and generally try to stay earth bound. This is a hyperresponsiveness to vestibular stimulation.

In Down syndrome, both hyper- and hyporesponsiveness can be modified through repeated experiences that gradually become more difficult. This allows the child to adapt and respond appropriately to a variety of experiences. Programming can and should begin in infancy, though even older children will usually respond favorably.

Neuromotor

The neuromotor problems that affect motor development in children with Down syndrome are hypotonia and decreased strength. The degree of hypotonia ranges from mild to severe. Muscle tone in children with Down syndrome is thought to improve with age. Hypotonia is usually combined with laxity of the ligaments around the joints. This causes excessive mobility of joints because the ligaments do not provide adequate stability.

Weakness is a significant problem for the child with Down syndrome. The muscles that flex tend to be weaker than the muscles that extend. Most flexors are located on the front of the body and cause joints to bend. The extensors are primarily found on the back of the body and cause joints to straighten. Weakness of the flexor muscles of the neck and trunk causes the infant to have difficulty lifting the head when pulled to sit. Also because the flexors of the trunk are weak, the infant often arches the back when being carried upright or when lying on the stomach.

Strength provides endurance or the ability to sustain a posture or movement for an extended period of time. Children with Down syndrome tire more quickly than other children and often participate in gross motor tasks for shortened periods of time. They may prefer to sit rather than stand and, though they are able to sit with a straight back, will quickly revert to sitting in a slumped posture, which requires less strength and endurance to maintain.

GROSS MOTOR INTERVENTION

Programming for the infant with Down syndrome should begin as soon as the diagnosis has been established and the family is ready to receive help. This may occur soon after delivery, particularly if the baby is having problems nippling to feed. General early intervention strategies are discussed in Chapter 9.

The intervention strategies for gross motor development discussed in this chapter are based on theories of neurodevelopment and sensory integration as well as infant behavior and learning. Within this context, the child with Down syndrome is guided toward the acquisition of those milestones that occur in normal gross motor development. The achievement of quality movement is considered of greater importance rather than pushing the child to perform motor milestones as quickly as possible.

Early Infancy

During the newborn period, the primary focus of gross motor programming is on handling, positioning, and strengthening. *Handling* is the term for the methods used to hold, lift, and carry a baby and includes diapering, feeding, dressing, and bathing. *Positioning* refers to techniques for placing and supporting an infant in a posture that enhances function, strength, or joint alignment. This includes individualized adaptation of equipment as well as modification of the environment. Handling and positioning are a component of the gross motor program well into childhood.

Positioning

The positions used with infants are lying on the stomach, back, side, and sitting. When babies are on their stomach, a folded towel or small wedge may be placed under their chest to help raise the head and position the arms in front of the body. Learning to visually attend can be encouraged by placing a bright interesting toy about 10–12 inches in front of the child (Fig. 7–1). Once infants are able to consistently maintain the upright position of the head with arms forward, use of the towel or wedge can be gradually discontinued. Toys can begin to be placed forward and slightly to each side to encourage the children to reach for them.

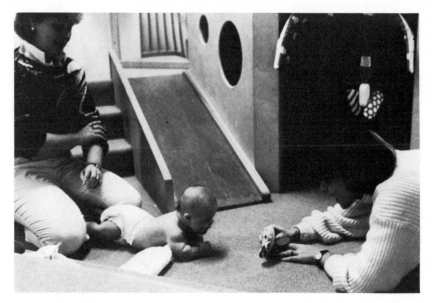

Figure 7-1. A child in the prone position being visually stimulated.

When lying on their backs, the babies may require support for the head, shoulders, and legs. A towel or blanket roll can be placed behind the back of the head so that it is tipped forward into slight neck flexion. A folded towel beneath the shoulders assists in raising the arms off the supporting surface. The babies are then able to bring their hands together on their chest for grasping and transferring toys from hand to hand. Swiping with the arms and reaching are also enhanced by support with the shoulders (Fig. 7-2). Towels may also be placed beside and slightly under the thighs to keep the legs from rolling out into the frog position to keep the babies from lying flat on the mattress.

Side-lying is a position that encourages early visual attending and object manipulation. It is also a foundation for rolling. In this position, the chin should be tucked forward into neck flexion and the arms and legs brought close together. Gravity assists the upper arm and leg during movement. To stay in this position, children must use both flexors and extensors of the neck, trunk, and hips. Initially, infants will require support behind the back with a roll, a pillow, crib bumper pads, or the commercially available crib cuddler. They will also need to have a small pillow placed under their head. With the children's increasing strength, these assists can be discontinued.

A variety of pieces of equipment, including car, feeder, and infant seats, can be used for supported sitting. These can be adapted by placing rolls behind the head and shoulders and beside the legs. The infants are

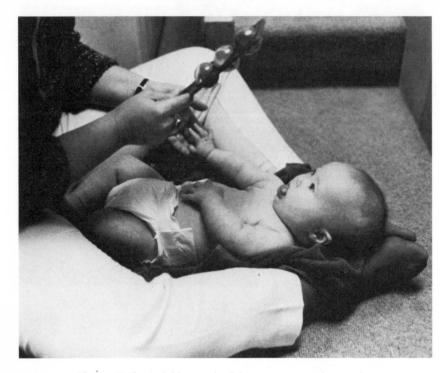

Figure 7-2. A child on its back being encouraged to reach.

gradually moved toward an upright, vertical position as head and trunk control improves. A commercially available plastic crate padded with towels can be used to support upright sitting (Fig. 7-3). A tray providing arm support will encourage reaching and playing with toys.

When sleeping, the legs should be positioned so that they do not lie flat on the mattress with the hips and knees bent in a frog position. This is done by placing rolls beside the thighs, by narrowing sleeping sacs by taking a larger side seam, or by gripping the legs of sleepers together. More aggressive approaches, such as wrapping the legs together, should be used only after consultation with a therapist or physician who can determine that the hip joints are developing correctly.

Handling

There are several carrying techniques appropriate for use with infants who have Down syndrome. Babies can be held at the parent's shoulder with the trunk and leg in extension. Or infants can be carried by positioning them in a forward-sitting posture while they are held at the

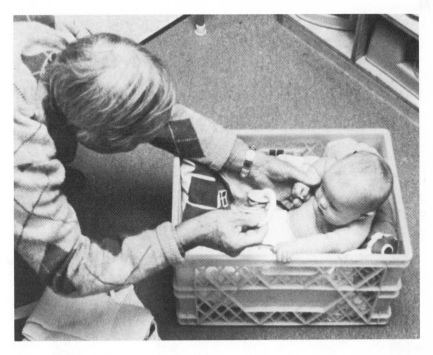

Figure 7-3. A padded plastic crate used to encourage upright sitting.

caregiver's side (Fig. 7-4). These are much better than the straddling "hip carry," which places the legs in a marked frog position. When holding infants cradled in the arms, the babies' head should be slightly flexed and the arms and legs close together.

The shaped (cut-out) commercial diaper encourages a more normal position of the legs by reducing the amount of material between the legs. Cloth diapers can be twisted in front to achieve the same goal. Preemie-size disposable diapers often are the best fit for the newborn.

The infant with Down syndrome should be positioned with the head and legs bent while being bathed. Commercially available inflatable plastic rings are often quite helpful in supporting the flexed posture. These provide security and allow the infant to relax and enjoy being bathed. This also frees the parent's hands for play and tactile stimulation.

Strengthening and Movement

In early infancy, strengthening begins with activating muscle groups. Of particular importance are the muscles of the neck and trunk as well as those of the shoulder and pelvic girdle. These are large, heavy work

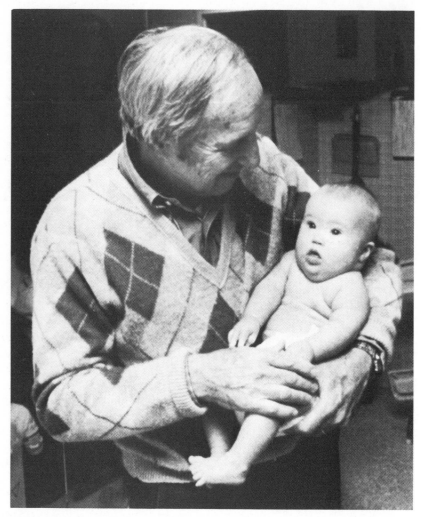

Figure 7–4. An infant being carried in a forward-sitting posture.

muscles, which provide the stability needed for controlled movement of the arms and legs. Babies with Down syndrome often need to be supported by surfaces and to work with gravity to increase their range of active movement. As strength increases, pushing away from the surface and acting against gravity for longer periods of time is encouraged.

Strengthening to gain head control is often begun in the vertical position. When carrying babies upright at the shoulder, parents should gradually reduce the amount of support they provide by lowering their hands on the babies' trunk. A method used to strengthen the flexors begins by holding infants at their chest in a supported sitting position. The babies are then very slowly tipped backwards until they appear to be losing the ability to hold the head forward. At this point, they are slowly returned to upright. The head should never be allowed to fall backwards into extension because of the potential presence of atlantoaxial instability. For the same reason, pull-to-sit should not be used until the child can maintain the head in alignment with the trunk throughout the movement.

Another strengthening technique begins in the supported sitting position previously described. The infants are very slowly tipped from side to side while they maintain their head in the upright position. It helps the babies to keep the head in position if the adult is in front and looking and talking to them while they are slowly tipped. Additional strengthening of the neck and upper trunk musculature can be facilitated while children are lying on the back or sitting with support. Once children are correctly positioned, they are encouraged to turn their head as they follow a toy with their eyes that is slowly being moved from side to side.

While lying on the stomach, babies use the neck and trunk extensor muscles for head and upper trunk lifting. A wedge under the chest provides support as infants are developing the ability to lift and extend the trunk and shoulder, while using the arms to hold up their weight. This often begins with the arms straight (extended). Later, infants will support themselves in prone with their elbows bent, bearing weight on their forearms. Securely holding the infants' buttocks often enhances head raising and weight bearing. Once infants are stable in prone weight bearing, they usually begin moving in a circular fashion (pivoting). Circular movement can be encouraged by placing toys just barely out of reach to the side.

Rolling usually begins from stomach to back, and starts after children can lift their head and push on extended arms. However, it is rolling from back to stomach that receives emphasis during gross motor programming. This is more difficult to achieve and requires the use of neck, arm, and hip flexors. Beginning in back lying, the arm that will be crossing the body is physically assisted forward so that it participates in the movement pattern rather than lagging behind the body. Later, reaching for a toy is used to encourage active incorporation of the arm into the movement. Initially, the top leg may need to be flexed at the hip and knee and slightly turned in the direction of the roll to assist the infant in the movement. Once rolling from back to stomach has developed, the leg is held so that it moves as the last portion of the pattern.

Middle Infancy

This period of development is characterized by increasing movement while on the stomach. The child with Down syndrome learns to creep on hands and knees, to move into and out of sitting, and to pull-to-stand.

Additionally, they are able to sit on the floor without help and to start standing with support.

Positioning

The desired position for sitting on the floor is with the back straight and weight on the buttocks. The legs should be extended forward with knees only slightly bent and fairly close together. Sitting with the legs in a circle and the ankles crossed (ring sitting) should be avoided as it exaggerates the knees out (frog) position of the legs. This causes children to sit with their weight shifted backwards onto their low back and results in rounding of the back and hyperextension or stacking of the head.

When children with Down syndrome begin to prop-sit on the floor, they will need to use either their legs or a raised surface for support because their arms are usually too short to reach the floor. A low bench or bed tray can be used. Back support in sitting can be achieved with a small ''legless'' chair (floor sitter) to which a strap that fits over the pelvis has been attached. The pelvic strap should cross the hip joint following the crease line of the hip. The strap should not be around the waist or trunk. Its purpose is to stabilize the pelvis, thereby providing the additional support needed to move and hold the arms in many positions during play.

When beginning to sit in a chair, the child with Down syndrome needs a chair of proper height and seat depth. The feet should be flat on the floor or a foot rest. The depth of the seat from the chair back should be such that the back of the knees are at the front edge of the chair. A small molded plastic booster seat or a wooden chair that converts to a step stool are usually satisfactory as a first chair. Firm inserts (styrofoam, wood, phone books) may need to be added to commercial child-sized chairs to limit both the width and depth. The seat of high chairs will need to be narrowed to keep the legs straight and to avoid ring sitting. The cloth-covered wing-back high chairs are preferred because they enhance the forward position of the arms, and the seat is not as deep as in most high chairs.

Strengthening and Movement

During this period, it is important to continue working on strengthening trunk flexors and extensors in supine and prone and to strengthen trunk rotation during rolling. As the child progresses toward the achievement of independent sitting, the correct movement between sitting and lying on the stomach should begin to be emphasized. While sitting on the floor, the child is helped to twist or rotate the trunk by guiding both hands so that they can be placed on the floor at one side of the body. One or both knees should be bent, pointing toward the hands. From this side-sitting position, children can move from sitting by lowering themselves onto their stomachs. This same pattern is reversed to come from prone to side-lying and up to sit. As children gain strength, they will require less physical assistance until they can perform the movement independently (Fig. 7–5). This rotational movement from sit to prone is used to avoid the tendency of children with Down syndrome to widely spread the legs to each side and lower or raise themselves straight forward onto or up from the stomach.

As children gain the skills necessary for independent sitting, protective extension of the arm is facilitated. In this reflex, the arms quickly extend to interrupt a fall and protect the body. To stimulate protective extension, the parents should begin by holding their children firmly at the hips in an upright position with their children's backs against their chests. From about 2 feet above the floor, they should tip their children forward so they are lowered head first toward the supporting surface. Initially, move the

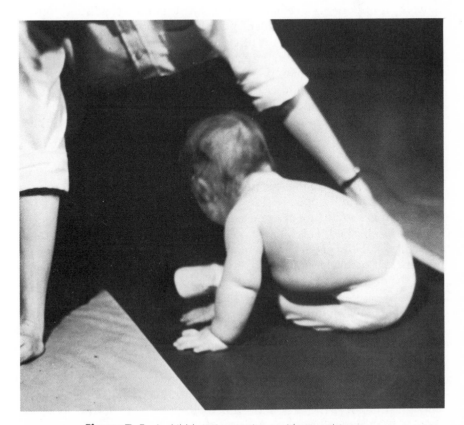

Figure 7–5. A child learning to sit up without assistance.

children slowly both forward and to each side to allow ample time for the response. As the children begin to extend their arms, the speed of movement can be increased. Protective extension can also be practiced while the children are sitting on the floor, in an armless chair, or on a bench by tipping them from side to side.

Often, belly-crawling precedes creeping on hands and knees and is the first efficient means of moving forward. When crawling on the stomach, the knees should be close to and somewhat under the body so that the leg and foot can be used to push the body forward. Tying children's shoelaces together so their feet can only spread 8–10 inches frequently helps to achieve this position. The arms need to be near the trunk with the elbows under the shoulders so that effective forward pulling occurs. As the children gain independence in crawling on the stomach, it is important to begin working on creeping (stomach up).

Creeping on hands and knees is often the most difficult developmental milestone to achieve for children with Down syndrome. However, with consistency and patience on the part of parents, most children will creep. This is an important developmental task as it plays a significant role in strengthening the trunk, shoulder, and pelvis girdles and in shifting weight from one side of the body to the other. During this period of skill development, emphasis should be on the achievement of a quality creeping pattern even though the child may prefer to stand.

Lower extremity weight bearing and weight shift are prerequisites for balancing on hands and knees and creeping with the stomach off the surface. Initially, it may be necessary to place babies over a roll to support the trunk and help maintain them in hands-and-knees position. Once the children can support themselves on hands and knees, they should be assisted in rocking forward and backward, then side to side. Reaching for a toy in front and to the side further develops strength and encourages weight shift to the opposite side of the body.

Walking should not be praised or encouraged until creeping has become established. This allows time for children to gain the strength and structural stability needed to maintain good alignment of the joints when walking. Of particular importance is the stability of the knees, ankles, and feet. The desired position for supported standing is one in which the hips are nearly straight and the knees slightly bent. There should be active movement between flexion and extension in both the hips and knees. The knees should not be locked stiffly into extension. For this reason, baby walkers are discouraged because they often encourage standing and moving with the hips bent and the knees in excessive extension.

Emphasis should continue to be on increasing the strength of the neck, trunk, and hip flexors. Assisted sit-ups are introduced once children have enough strength in the neck and trunk to hold the head in straight alignment with the body during the movement. Lying on the back and reaching to knees and feet also strengthens flexors. Babies can play "body parts" and "look here" games. During these lying-on-the-back and reaching-forward tasks, the knees should be 4–5 inches apart and the buttocks rolled up and off the supporting surface.

Sensory Activities

Sensory activities that stimulate awareness or modify tolerance to touch and movement are introduced at this time. Particular attention is directed to the tactile system and the tolerance of the hands, face, and mouth to a variety of textures. These can include texture balls for play, foamy soap for the bath, and body rubs with lotion, terry cloth, or a soft sponge.

A variety of movement experiences, including swinging in the parent's arms and participating in gentle roughhousing, as well as being moved in carts or wagons should be provided. If frightened, children should not be forced but gently assisted in gradually moving from resistance to tolerance and finally to achieving active initiation and participation.

Late Infancy

It is during this phase of development that children with Down syndrome refine their skill on hands and knees and become efficient creepers. They begin to stand independently and step along furniture. The culmination of this period is independent walking.

Strengthening and Movement

Creeping with the knees positioned directly under the hips and the hands under the shoulders is emphasized. Creeping through tunnels or within a narrow space is often helpful. Obstacle courses can be used to challenge the balance and strength. They can include creeping over low objects, up-and-down inclines, and through barrels.

The transitional movements used to get from one position to another are important in increasing strength and improving balance. A necessary component of transitional movement is the ability to twist the trunk while either the shoulders or pelvis remains fixed (trunk rotation). This is often difficult for children with Down syndrome but is important because it is necessary for fluid and efficient movement. An activity than enhances trunk rotation is sitting or standing with the pelvis stabilized while reaching with both hands for toys that have been placed to either side. Active rotation continues to be facilitated during rolling as well as during movement from hands and knees to side sitting. It is usually necessary at first to stabilize the legs and pelvis to gain the desired rotation.

When children begin to pull themselves up to standing, they should learn to get up using half-kneeling rather than pushing up with both legs extending at the same time. Beginning from kneeling, one leg is brought forward so the hip and knee are at 90° of flexion and the foot is flat on the floor. Children are assisted to push-to-stand using the flexed leg while pulling with their arms (Fig. 7–6). At this time in development, the most common method of moving from standing to the floor for children with Down syndrome is to fall backwards into sit. Physical assistance may be necessary to help children gain the ability to lower themselves to the floor with bent knees.

Initially, a mid-chest-height surface will be needed for supported standing. As children are able to stand more securely and balance while playing with toys, the height of the supporting surface should be lowered. The hips should remain extended and the knees slightly flexed. The surface should not be so low that they are able to lean forward with the

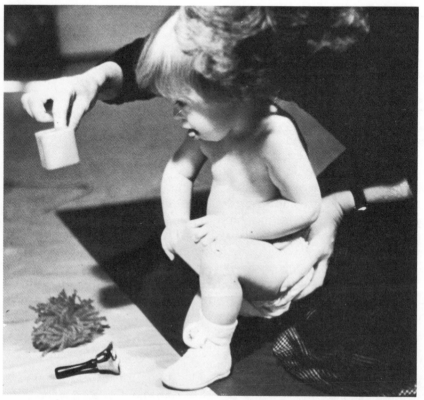

Figure 7–6. Encouraging a child to stand from the half-kneeling position.

hips flexed and support their weight on the trunk. As balance in standing increases, children will begin to push away from the support.

Parents should observe their children's standing posture, particularly checking the position of the feet and the knees. The feet should not be rolled inward nor should the knees be locked in extension. Many children with Down syndrome will stand and walk more securely if they are fitted with sturdy high-top shoes. Parents may wish to have their children evaluated to determine whether shoe modifications or fabricated inserts are indicated.

Cruising is walking sideways while holding onto something in easy reach. When children cruise, they bear weight on one leg as they take a sideways step with the other leg. This movement can be facilitated by holding children at the pelvis and shifting their weight onto one leg. Toys are placed to the side and slightly out of reach to stimulate movement. If the step is too large, the moving leg may need to be somewhat restrained.

Once children with Down syndrome are cruising efficiently along and around objects, it is time to encourage movement between pieces of furniture. At first, children will only reach with their arms, but eventually they will begin to take steps. Once stepping between objects begins, the distance between them is gradually increased. At the same time, walking forward is begun by pushing large, stable objects, often kitchen chairs or weighted push toys.

Children with Down syndrome often take their first steps while positioned in supported standing. Support may be provided by a wall, a person, or a piece of furniture. At this stage, children tend to fall forward into a waiting person's arms. Early walking is usually done with stiff legs, and weight bearing is on the heel of the foot. Gradually, the center of gravity shifts forward so that weight bearing occurs across the whole foot and the feet become closer together.

Parents need to be aware of the position of the arms when their children are walking; they should be down by the sides and fairly close to the body. Though the pattern of holding the arms up and away from the body is one usually observed in early toddling, it is discouraged in children with Down syndrome because of their tendency to exaggerate the arm posture and prolong its use. Carrying weighted objects such as plastic syrup bottles partially filled with sand or water assists in bringing the arms down and in developing arm swing.

As children gain security in walking, activities that challenge the balance in standing are introduced. These include walking on slightly soft or uneven surfaces such as mats and up-and-down inclines. Also, boards can be used that are designed to supply some challenge for the upright position (tilt boards). As balance and pelvic girdle strength improve, the widened position of the legs will continue to narrow.

The muscles that flex the neck, trunk, and hip as well as muscles that rotate the trunk continue to require strengthening. Physically assisted sit-ups should now incorporate trunk rotation as the children reach for the left foot with the right hand and vice versa. Control of the muscles around the hip is enhanced by creeping up and down inclines and over objects as well as moving slowly from sitting to standing and back to sitting. Additionally, coming to stand through half-kneel and supported movement between standing and squatting can be incorporated into play (Fig. 7-7).

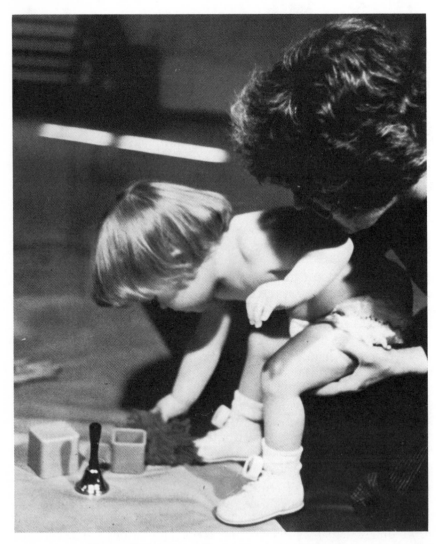

Figure 7-7. Incorporating learning to stand with play.

Sensory Activities

Sensory discrimination continues to be an important component of play. A wide variety of tactile activities should be introduced including water and sand tables. Materials such as aquarium gravel, beans, rice, and eggshells as well as finger paint, lotion, and shaving cream can be used. Forceful pressing, squeezing, and patting are primary components of these tasks. It is during this phase of development that resistance to handling materials as well as foods may become apparent. This occurs most often with textures that are somewhat soft and slick.

Movement activities should provide a wide variety of experiences and include raised and moving surfaces such as swings, riding toys, suspended platforms or tires, blanket or towel swings, and seesaws. Children with Down syndrome should be encouraged to creep and walk over uneven or unsteady surfaces such as ramps, water beds, suspended bridges, and sand piles.

Early Childhood

During this stage of development, sitting, walking, and climbing skills are further refined. Running, jumping, and stair climbing begin as well as kicking, rolling, and throwing both large and small balls.

Positioning

Sitting patterns continue to be monitored and enhanced since children often spend considerable time playing on the floor. The desired posture for floor sitting is still one in which the back is straight and weight bearing occurs on the buttocks. The patterns most recommended are sitting with legs extended in front and side-sitting with knees bent and legs together on one side. Cross-legged sitting is discouraged because the widened base of support decreases the opportunity to use balance reactions and tends to cause children to sit with rounded backs.

Chair and table heights usually need to be adapted to accommodate the shortened stature of children with Down syndrome. Both the height and depth of small chairs must be modified so that children can sit with their feet on the floor and their backs supported. Tables usually need to be lowered so that they are at an appropriate height for feeding and hand activities. Rectangular rather than round tables are best because they provide more surface for arm support.

Toilet training may begin at this time, and the potty chair selected should be of acceptable depth and width. The commercially available single unit molded plastic potty seat provides good support and is easy for children to get on and off independently.

Strengthening and Movement

Control is gradually increasing in standing and in intermediary postures. Kneeling with the hips straight is often observed spontaneously during play. Walking in this position while pushing a small mobile object is used to strengthen the pelvic girdle and improve balance. As independence in knee walking is gained, this movement can be incorporated into obstacle courses.

Children will now squat during play. Squatting is most frequently used to pick up or place objects on the floor. This requires slow, controlled movement and balanced strength of the muscles of the trunk, hips, and knees. Children may initially need to be supported at the pelvis to maintain the buttocks in a position higher than the knees. Movement in and out of squat can be used during imitation games or group songs. Eventually it should become a component of spontaneous movement and play.

The development of heel-toe walking as well as running and jumping is dependent on the ability to push the body forward with the ball of the foot. This forceful propulsion is needed to develop for forward and upward movement. A small jogging trampoline that is not too taut is effective in training jumping. Adults stand behind the children on the trampoline and apply downward pressure through the shoulders as the trampoline is bounced. Once the youngsters are able to jump on the trampoline with both feet pushing off at the same time, they are ready to begin to attempt jumping down from a surface such as a low bench or a low step. The children's hands are held, and they are gently pulled forward at push-off. It may be necessary to explain and demonstrate the bent position of the knees. Jumping on the floor is more difficult than either trampoline or downward jumping. It sometimes helps to use a slightly springy surface, such as a foam rubber mattress.

It is best to introduce stair climbing using nonstandard stairs that are smaller in height and depth and have steps with solid, closed backs rather than open ones. Ideally, stairs should be narrow enough that both hand rails can be used. The pelvic girdle control needed for balance and foot placement during stair climbing can be practiced by stepping up onto and off of low objects such as stools and playground stepping stones. Gradually the reliance on rails should be reduced and children should be taught to alternate their feet when stepping.

Balance in walking is enhanced by providing activities that require walking on a narrow surface, such as 6–8-inch-wide balance beams or railroad ties found in the playground or park. Other tasks include stepping through the rungs of a ladder, over low hurdles, or in and out of small hoops that have been placed on the floor. These activities can be gradually made more difficult by raising the board, ladder, or hoops off the floor.

Children with Down syndrome do better at kicking and throwing a ball than catching. A large ball is used for two-handed overhand throwing. This requires shoulder and arm strength and control. Initially, children may throw almost straight down, but they should be encouraged to aim for targets at gradually increasing distances. Most children need to be shown how to position their hands and arms for catching. In the beginning, the arms tend to trap the ball against the body. Later, the hands begin to be used. It is most difficult to catch a ball when movement of the hands, arm, or body is necessary in order to be in the right position.

Kicking requires the ability to balance on one foot while shifting weight. At first, children will run and randomly kick the ball. However, once they are able to stand on one foot long enough to kick a placed ball, they should be guided to kick the ball forward toward a target, such as a portable soccer goal or a large box.

Sensory Activities

Tactile activities begin to include the differentiation of textures, shapes, and surfaces. Familiar objects can be buried in sand, water, cotton balls, or styrofoam packing material to be located through the sense of touch. Tactile boxes, feely bags, and water play are used to introduce the properties of soft, hard, hot, and cold. Art activities include collages and forms that require spatial organization. Localization and identification of body parts become more precise.

Playgrounds should provide a variety of movement experiences. While being monitored for safety, children with Down syndrome should be encouraged to climb, slide, swing, and spin. This includes hanging from the knees or swinging by the arms from a low monkey bar or a trapeze. Tricycles may need the foot pedals raised. Riding down a slight incline assists the child with propulsion when learning to pedal.

CONCLUSION

It is no doubt apparent to the reader that considerable time and effort could be invested in enhancing the gross motor skills of the child with Down syndrome. Many may wonder if this is time well spent. What should a parent hope to achieve?

It has been the experience of the authors that children with Down syndrome who have participated in gross motor programs during infancy and childhood are considerably more appropriate in appearance and better able to interact and participate with their peers. They have improved posture and more fluid movement patterns. Many of the avoidance behaviors associated with sensory hypersensitivity become extinguished and, consequently, interaction and mastery of the environment are enhanced.

A potential benefit from a good gross motor foundation is a broader range of opportunities provided for both work and play. As their world expands and a greater variety of opportunities occurs, children with Down syndrome are then better prepared to meet the challenge if they have gained the skill and self-confidence that motor proficiency brings.

REFERENCES

Caplan, F., & Caplan, T. (1973a). *The first twelve months of life.* New York: Grossett & Dunlap.

Caplan, F., & Caplan, T. (1973b). *The power of play.* New York: Anchor Press/Doubleday.

Caplan, F., & Caplan, T. (1977). *The second twelve months of life.* New York: Grossett & Dunlap.

Chandler, L., et al. (1980). *Movement assessment in infants.* Washington, DC.

Connolly, B., Morgan, S., Russell, F.F., & Richardson, B. (1976). Early intervention with Down syndrome children. *Physical Therapy, 60*(11), 1405–1408.

Connolly, B., & Russell, F. (1976). Interdisciplinary early intervention program. *Physical Therapy, 56*(2), 155–158.

Connor, F.P., et al. (1978). *Program guide for infants and toddlers with neuro-motor and other developmental disabilities.* New York: Teachers' College Press.

Cunningham, C.C. (1982). *Down's syndrome: An introduction for parents.* London: Souvenir Press.

Diamond, L.S., Lynn, D., & Sigman, B. (1981). Orthopedic disorders in patients with Down's syndrome. *Orthopedic Clinics of North America, 12*(1).

Domitriev, V. (1982). *Time to begin.* Washington: Caring, Inc.

Furuno, S., et al. (1979). *HELP, Hawaii early learning profile activity guide.* Palo Alto, CA: VORT Corporation.

Gibson, D. (1978). *Down syndrome, the psychology of mongolism.* New York: Cambridge University Press.

Gilfoyle, E., & Grady, A. (1981). *Children adapt.* Thorofare, NJ: Slack.

Gordon, I.J. (1975). *The infant experience.* Westerville, OH: Merrill.

Hanson, M.J. (1987). *Teaching the infant with Down syndrome: A guide for parents and professionals.* Austin, TX: Pro-Ed.

Harris, S. (1981). Effects of neurodevelopmental therapy on motor performance of infants with Down's syndrome. *Developmental Medicine and Child Neurology, 23,* 477–483.

Henderson, S.E., Morris, J., & Frith, U. (1981). The motor deficit in Down's syndrome children: A problem of timing? *Journal of Child Psychology and Psychiatry, 22,* 233–245.

Holt, K.S. (1975). *Movement and child development.* Philadelphia: Lippincott.

Illingsworth, R.S. (1974). *The development of the infant and young child, normal and abnormal.* London: Churchill Livingston.

Kerr, R., et al. (1985). Motor skill acquisition by individuals with Down syndrome. *American Journal of Mental Deficiency, 90*(3), 313–318.

Lane, D., & Stratford, B. (1985). *Current approaches to Down's syndrome.* New York: Praeger Special Studies.

Montague, A. (1971). *Touching.* New York: Harper & Row.

Piper, M.C., & Pless, I.B. (1980). Early intervention for infants with Down's syndrome: A controlled trial. *Pediatrics, 65,* 463–468.

Pueschel, S.M. (1984). *The young child with Down syndrome.* New York: Human Sciences Press.

Pueschel, S.M., et al. (1987). *New perspectives on Down syndrome.* Baltimore: Brookes.

Pueschel, S.M., et al. (1982). *Down syndrome: Advances in biomedicine and the behavioral sciences.* Massachusetts: The Ware Press.

Pueschel, S.M. (Ed.). (1981). *Down syndrome: Growing and learning.* New York: Andres & McMeel.

Rast, M.M., et al. (1985). Motor control in infants with Down syndrome. *Developmental Medicine and Child Neurology, 27*(5), 682–685.

Sleight, D., & Niman-Reed, C. (1984). *Gross motor and oral motor development in children with Down syndrome: Birth through three years.* St. Louis, MO: St. Louis Association for Retarded Citizens.

White, B. (1975). *The first three years of life.* Englewood Cliffs, NJ: Prentice-Hall.

GLOSSARY

Adaptive equipment: specially designed or modified equipment used to meet a child's specific postural needs

Balance: ability to maintain a position when the center of gravity is displaced

Crawling: forward movement of the child while on the stomach

Creeping: forward movement of the child while on hands and knees

Depressed: less than expected

Extensors: muscles that extend or straighten joints, usually located on the back of the body

Flexors: muscles that flex or bend joints, usually located on the front of the body

Floppy: hypermobile with low muscle tone

Gross motor: primarily requiring the larger muscles of the trunk, shoulder, and pelvic girdle; used for head control, creeping, sitting, standing, and walking

Handling: techniques for holding and moving that are specifically designed to help the child experience more normal tone, posture, and movement

Hypersensitivity: excessive response to sensory stimulation

Hyposensitivity: abnormally decreased response to sensory stimulation

Hypotonia: decreased muscle tone

Pelvic girdle: area of the trunk including the lower trunk and hips

Prone: lying on the stomach

Proprioception: internal awareness of joint movement, including that from range, direction, and speed

Range of motion: the amount of movement that is possible at a joint.

Rotation: twisting movement of the trunk occurring in a horizontal plane between the hips and shoulders

Sensory motor: pertaining to the combined function of sensory systems and motor mechanisms

Shoulder girdle: area of the trunk including the scapula, upper trunk, and shoulder joints

Supine: lying on the back

Tactually defensive: resisting, avoiding, or rejecting nonthreatening touch

Tone, muscle: amount of tension present in a muscle

Vestibular system: the sensory system that influences balance, posture, and locomotion

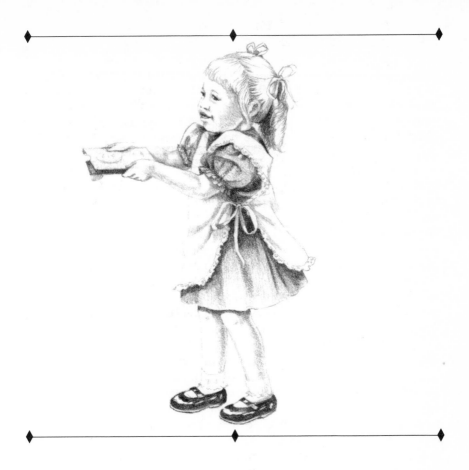

CHAPTER EIGHT

FACILITATING SPEECH AND LANGUAGE DEVELOPMENT

JON F. MILLER

Paul is 5 years old. He is a very active boy who communicates with sign language as well as with speech. He talks mostly about the activities and people around him in two- and three-word sentences. He is a lively communicator, speaking freely to strangers and family alike. His speech, however, is very difficult to understand for those not familiar with him. Jennifer is 20 months old, is beginning to pull herself up on the furniture, and is walking with support. She makes some speech sounds in response to her parents, brothers, and sisters talking to her. She uses gestures and vocalizations to communicate with her family, expressing her desire for something to eat, something to drink, or someone to stop what they are doing. Her family knows what she means, but strangers do not. William is 12 years old and involved in a variety of school activities. He is a Special Olympian, participating in track and field. He likes school, particularly activities having to do with art, drawing, and clay. He talks about present activities as well as those activities in which he has participated in the past. He primarily talks in four- and five-word sentences, and he is able to communicate relationships between past activities and the present. Most people can understand William's speech, though when he gets excited, those not familiar with him find him difficult to understand.

All of these children share a common characteristic—they all have Down syndrome. They also all have communication skills that allow them to share basic feelings and to express wants and desires with those around them. Their communication skills, however, are not as advanced as other aspects of their development. This particular characteristic of these children is a great puzzle to scientists working in the area of child development, language development, and development of intelligence. It would appear that these children, for a variety of reasons, do not communicate as well as would be expected.

This chapter briefly reviews what is known about language and communication in children with Down syndrome and discusses some ways in which language and communication development for people with Down syndrome can be promoted.

LANGUAGE DEVELOPMENT

Written descriptions of research clearly specify the major components necessary to develop communication skills and learn a language. First, there are a variety of skills and abilities that the individual brings to the

Work on this paper was supported in part by a research grant from the National March of Dimes (#12-197) and from core research support to the Waisman Center on Mental Retardation and Human Development, University of Wisconsin, Madison, for the NIH, NICHD, Mental Retardation Research Centers Program.

language learning task, including basic cognitive, sensory, and perceptual skills. Basic cognitive skills include those that make it possible to acquire knowledge of the world and the ability to recognize and remember events and people. Some researchers believe that human beings are particularly equipped to learn a language with great ease without requiring planned instruction. For example, children without learning problems retain some aspects of the meaning of a new word upon hearing it only once. Nondelayed children after about 18 months of age learn five to seven new words every day. Whether or not human beings have special cognitive skills for language learning has been the subject of considerable debate. It is, however, an important point for us to consider as we evaluate the language learning characteristics of children with Down syndrome. We will need to consider the possibility that deficits in these special language learning skills interact with general intellectual abilities to cause increased communication difficulties.

The second major contributing factor to language learning is, of course, the environment. In order to learn language, children must first hear a language spoken around them. Then they must participate with other human beings in speaking that language. The people in each child's environment must be responsive to that child's communicative attempts; e.g., they must continue to point out the names of objects, actions, and relations in the child's ongoing activities. As we consider what we can do to facilitate language and communication in children with Down syndrome, it is clear that the most productive procedure is to manipulate the environmental characteristics in hopes of provoking the most effective use of the child's language learning skills. We want to be able to organize the child's environment to maximize the ability to acquire new communication skills through everyday experience.

LANGUAGE SKILLS OF CHILDREN WITH DOWN SYNDROME

There are a number of reasons why children with Down syndrome are likely to have problems in learning basic language and communication skills (Miller, 1987). First, there is increased frequency of middle ear infection, which is frequently associated with delayed language. Frequent middle ear infections can result in hearing loss, which can affect the level at which children are able to hear a language spoken around them. Second, there may be deficits in the ability to move the speech system, particularly in coordinating the rapid movements of the tongue, lips, jaw, and palate, with voicing and respiration. There is increasing evidence that this motor difficulty impairs the ability to produce intelligible speech in children with Down syndrome. Third, there is increasing evidence to suggest that children with Down syndrome may have language learning problems that are beyond those commonly associated with slow development. That is, there may be deficits in specific cognitive skills necessary for language learning. Fourth, and most important for continued language learning, is that as children get older, there appear to be increasing deficits in language and communication skills relative to other abilities. At the same time, there appear to be decreased expectations for communication performance of these children—i.e., less communication is expected of them as they get older. Family members may not talk to them as much and may expect less talk in return; therefore, the children are deprived of communicative practice. The result is limited opportunity to acquire new vocabulary and to practice those language skills that they do have in social situations. Children with Down syndrome begin the language learning process with a number of concerns, which need to be attended to in order to promote language learning.

EARLY LANGUAGE LEARNING

Children with Down syndrome, in general, develop an ability to understand language and to produce language at rates that are consistent with their general intellectual abilities through the first 3–4 years of age. After this time, it appears that language development continues but not at the same rate as other intellectual abilities. This may be due to any of the four factors mentioned above or to some other factors that are unidentified as yet. In order to understand this change in rate of development, it is important to understand that language is a very complex system, made up of a number of components. Children with Down syndrome are able to perform some components better than others. For example, in learning vocabulary—or the individual words that stand for objects, events, and actions—these children seem to do as well as their peers of equal mental age. In the area of using language for communicative purposes, as in determining when to talk and when not to talk and figuring out what's appropriate to say and what isn't in social situations, it appears that the children with Down syndrome do as well as would be expected at their mental age. In the area of grammar—or the combination of words into thoughts—however, children beyond the age of 3–4 years of age show increasing difficulties.

Development among components of language (i.e., vocabulary, grammar, and social use) is quite variable. Our overall understanding of child development, however, is limited by the nature of the studies that have been conducted to date. We have very few studies that have followed the same children for 3–5 years and reported the exact course of development. The more frequent approach is to study children for 1 or 2 years or to simply study different groups of children at different ages and report the observed differences as developmental changes. This is not an accurate way to describe the changes as they occur over time. It is safe to say at this juncture that children with Down syndrome are variable both in the course of their intellectual development and the course of their language and communication development.

To facilitate language, there are two primary considerations. The first is to develop speech skills to procure intelligible speech in a variety of situations. The second is learning the language system to represent objects, acts, actions, and relationships in their environment—that is, the words, the sentence structures, and the discourse skills necessary to communicate effectively. (These are discussed as independent characteristics in the section on facilitation strategies.) Finally, it is important to note that children at different ages will require different approaches. Activities for children up to 3 years of age include games, finger play, and redundant conversation about daily routines. Afterward, it is necessary to note how the child changes and how the child's communication needs change in order to continue to foster development. Older children and adults need interaction about life activities, but these must be things that are of interest to them and to others their age.

SUGGESTIONS FOR FACILITATING LANGUAGE AND COMMUNICATION SKILLS

In this section, two primary areas are considered. The first area concerns activities for facilitating the development of speech, with goals of improving the speech intelligibility. The second area is language as a system to represent the child's knowledge of the world. The language area includes working on vocabulary, grammar, and the range of meanings expressed by the child with words or with sentences. (For example, basic meanings include naming objects and actions, expressing location of objects and people, expressing causal relations, and expressing temporal relations among events.) The language area also includes learning the social use of language, as in using language to request, to express wants and needs, to make comments, to persuade and inform, to tell stories, and to engage in conversation in a variety of social situations.

This chapter presents some basic principles that can be useful in facilitating language growth in the child, by providing the child with a variety of opportunities in which to use language learning abilities. It is hoped that these principles can guide parents and teachers as they interact with the child who has Down syndrome.

As communicators we play two roles: speaker and listener. Each of us must be able to move back and forth between these when interacting with a conversational partner. Children's abilities to take these roles continue to develop over a long period of time throughout childhood. The first set of principles relates to the early periods of development; however, due to delays in development, the procedures may be useful for older children also.

Speech Goals for the Child

1. Increase the ability to respond to people and objects. The more we can promote people and object recognition, action, and response, the greater the opportunity for advancing communication skills. While responsiveness is an internal construct—that is, the product of the child's internal perceptual and conceptual abilities—it can be assumed that environmental influences can affect the child's opportunity and desire to respond.

2. Increase the frequency of vocal, verbal productions. Speech improvement will come with practice. The greater the speech output, the more opportunity for modifying the quality of speech. In order to improve movement patterns, the patterns must be practiced. Speech is a motor activity involving the careful coordination and timing of a number of activities including breathing, control of the larynx, and movements of the head, palate, tongue, lips, and jaw.

3. Increase production of sounds and the variety of sounds made. This includes two parts. The first is the sounds themselves, such as differentiating among bs and ps and ds and gs by using different parts of the speech system. The second has to do with characteristics such as speaking rate, intensity (how loud or soft), pitch, variation (in tone from high to low), and duration (how long speech can continue on a single breath). These characteristics contribute significantly to producing intelligible speech. They are controlled primarily by breathing and the laryngeal system, and improvements here will add greatly to the child's ability to produce more speech and more varied speech, aiding the listener to understand.

4. Making the transition from vocal behavior, creating sounds for self amusement, to using sounds to stand for objects and actions in the environment, e.g., saying words. It appears that many children with Down syndrome are trying to say words earlier than is recognized by persons in the child's environment, because their speech is difficult to understand and the words they use are simple labels rather than descriptive or action words. This is why sign language programs are often effective in helping children express words earlier and be understood when speech difficulties prevent producing words clearly.

Suggestions for Parents and Siblings

In order to introduce activities to promote change in performance, it is necessary to carefully observe that performance. There are two things that need to be observed and documented at the beginning. The first is to identify situations and activities throughout the day in which the child is most vocal. Every child is more vocal in some situations than others. For some it is during mealtime, for others, it's during bathing. For others still, it is while listening to music. Make a list of these situations over the course of a week or two, noting three things: a description of the situation itself, the length of time this situation continues, and how many times each of these situations occur during the day.

The second characteristic to be documented is how much the child responds to people and things by looking, touching, or playing during vocal situations as well as other situations. Responding is basic to communication. Without children taking note of their environment and responding to it, hopes of developing a communication system are greatly diminished. Some children are more responsive than others. It is possible to improve both vocalization and responsiveness skills by lengthening the amount of time children spend in these communication-enhancing contexts. This will do two things: (a) It will increase the frequency of the child's vocalizations by providing more practice; and (b) it will increase the opportunity for interaction with parents, siblings, and others. Under the conditions of maximal responsiveness, it is possible to introduce speech by talking to children about ongoing activities. It is important to use a variety of speech sounds and to vary the intensity and length of the utterances.

It is helpful to introduce music to children at an early age. Listening to music provides auditory stimulation, and children frequently respond with enthusiasm. Young children enjoy a variety of music types; some children prefer country and western, others rock and roll, and still others the classics. Expose children to several types of music so that they can select favorites.

Language activities should be a natural part of children's days. It is not appropriate to set aside special times of the day for working on speech and language. Communication cannot be learned in a formal lesson but must be part of the ongoing activity. During ordinary caregiving tasks, play with the child, talking about the objects of the play, and introduce interactive games such as "pat-a-cake" and "peek-a-boo" and "so big." These activities all have vocal initiation and responsiveness components to them, which are skills necessary to developing communication. The activities also promote turntaking and social interaction and responsiveness.

A speech-language pathologist can evaluate the child and suggest specific sound patterns or specific speech characteristics for the child to practice. Knowing the situations of frequent vocalizations and vocal characteristics of the child can provide the speech pathologist with valuable information needed to design a maximally effective program. The goal is simply to provide basic information on developing skills to facilitate language and communication. Specific concerns about a particular child's speech should be directed to a professional who has the opportunity to evaluate the child.

Facilitating Language and Communication Development

The distinction between speech sounds and language can be thought of developmentally. Children progress from producing a variety of speech sounds without intent to form words up to 10–12 months of age, at which time they combine those speech sounds and use them as words representing objects, actions, and relationships in the environment.

In order to understand the child's role in learning words through speech, it is necessary to draw the distinction between speech and language. First, it is important to note that children begin the learning process by understanding and producing a very few words in specific, frequently recurring situations. For example, they will understand and say their own name, names of family members, names of their pets, or names of favorite toys, but only in situations in which these people and objects are close by every day. After children are able to understand and, some time later, speak about 20 words, there occurs in children without Down syndrome a period of rapid learning of new words. We do not know as yet whether the same period of rapid vocabulary acquisition occurs in children with Down syndrome because we do not have studies that follow the same children during the first 3 years of life; we can speculate, however, that such a period should occur. It is important to note that children appear to acquire words more rapidly on their own, even when the language environment hasn't changed significantly. So there must be something children learn through the acquisition of 20 different words that leads them to acquire new words in a more efficient manner.

We cannot make children learn new words, but we can create a rich and stimulating environment in which they can come to understand that words stand for or represent people, objects, actions, and relationships in the environment. While we can teach children to imitate words, these words will not be used spontaneously with meaning unless children conceptualize them as representing something, rather than as just being a series of sounds. For example, children without Down syndrome between 6 and 8 months of age will frequently produce sounds such as "da-da" or "ma-ma," but they will not be producing these sounds as words, that is, as representing mother or father. At 12–15 months, however, these same sounds will be used to comment on mother or father entering a room or as a request for objects out of reach. At first, these sounds are produced as a kind of vocal play; later they come to have meaning in the earliest stages of communication development. In order to facilitate language and communication development, activities must be used that will lead children to come to understand that words do stand for objects and actions in the environment.

CHILD GOALS

The first goal is to increase the frequency of the child's communicative productions. These communicative acts are expressed in two ways initially: first, through gestures, and second, through vocal and verbal means. These are usually easily recognized by adults as communication expressing a variety of basic meanings. Initially, children express two basic communicative functions. First, they direct adults' attention to some event or object in their environment. The resulting attention is usually interpreted by the child as a communication response from the adult. The second function is the use of an adult as a means of obtaining objects or other goals, as in early requesting behavior. For example, the child standing in front of the refrigerator saying "ah, ah, ah" while pointing at the refrigerator door is certainly making an early request. Adults have little difficulty interpreting this as a request and will learn to understand if the request is for a favorite juice, or a glass of milk, or the leg of the Christmas turkey. Over time, children express their basic communicative intentions using words, which come to replace their early gestures. Research studies frequently find that children with Down syndrome tend to use gestures for a more prolonged period of time than do other children. There is some speculation that the prolonged use of gestures may be linked to difficulties in producing clear speech sounds.

As words enter the child's productive vocabulary, they represent a variety of objects, animals, toys, etc., that the child comes in contact with daily. Table 8–1 provides a list of the first 50 words produced by 18 children without Down syndrome in a longitudinal study conducted by Katherine Nelson. This vocabulary list can be used to help understand the variety of words children understand and produce. It is important to ask, what environment helped the child to learn each of these words? Then, situations in which the child will have an opportunity to learn these words

Table 8-1.

Fifty Early Words Used by Children

Category and Word	Frequency	Category and Word	Frequency
Food and drink		Frog	1
Juice	12	Goose	1
Milk	10	Monkey	1
Cookie	10	Moose	1
Water	8	Pig	1
Toast	7	Puppy	1
Apple	5	Tiger	1
Cake	5	Turkey	1
Banana	3	Turtle	1
Drink	3		
Bread	2	Eating and Drinking	
Butter	2	Utensils	
Cheese	2	Bottle	8
Egg	2	Cup	4
Pea(s)	2	Spoon	2
(Lolli)pop	2	Glass	1
Candy	1	Knife	1
Clackers	1	Fork	1
Coffee	1	Dish	1
Cracker	1	Tray	1
Food	1		
Gum	1	Clothing	
Meat	1	Shoes	11
Melon	1	Hat	5
Noodles	1	Socks	4
Nut	1	Boots	2
Peach	1	Belt	2
Pickle	1	Coat	2
Pizza	1	Tights	1
Soda	1	Slippers	1
Spaghetti	1	Shirt	1
		Dress	1
Animals		Bib	1
Dog (variants)	16		
Cat (variants)	14	Toys and Play	
Duck	8	Equipment	
Horse	5	Ball	13
Bear	4	Blocks	7
Bird	4	Doll	4
Cow (variants)	4	Teddy bear	2
Bee	1	Bike	2
Bug	1	Walker	1
Donkey	1	Swing	1

Category and Word	Frequency	Category and Word	Frequency
Vehicles		Watch	3
Car	13	Tissue	1
Boat	6	Chalk	1
Truck	6	Pen	1
Bus	2	Paper	1
Plane	1	Scissors	1
Choo-choo	1	Pocketbook	1
		Money	1
Furniture and			
Household Items		Outdoor Objects	
Clock	7	Snow	4
Light	6	Flower	2
Blanket	4	House	2
Chair	3	Moon	2
Door	3	Rock	2
Bed	1	Flag	1
Crib	1	Tree	1
Pillow	1	Map	1
Telephone	1		
Washing machine	1	Places	
Drawer	1	Pool	3
		Beach	1
Personal Items		School	1
Key	6	Porch	1
Book	5		

Nominals, grouped by semantic category, are present in the first 50-word vocabularies of 18 children. The digits to the right of each word represent the number of children using that word in Nelson's sample (1973). Adult form of word is used in this table, but many words had several variant forms, particularly the animal words.

From Nelson, K. (1973). Structure and strategy in learning to talk. *Monographs of the Society for Research in Child Development, 38*, 1–138. Copyright by the Society for Research in Child Development, Inc. Reprinted by permission.

can be designed. Table 8-2 provides a brief characterization of the developmental milestones of learning verbal language skills.

The onset of producing two words at a time signals the onset of the acquisition of grammar. Multiword expressions are used for a variety of relational meanings that are elaborated as children learn more and more about language. Children acquire the ability to talk about what they have seen and learned about their environment—that is, their knowledge of the world. The links between learning language and learning about the world are direct. Our expectation is that children with Down syndrome should be able to represent what they know about the world; anything

Table 8-2.
Developmental and Criterion-Referenced Scale for Identification
of Communication Deficits in the First 2 Years of Life

Physiological Behavioral Indices of Problem Status at Birth
    Feeding problems
    Weak cry
    Congenital anomalies
    Syndrome
    Orofacial anomalies
    Laryngeal anomalies
    Motor deficits (e.g., cerebral palsy)
    Low birth weight

Behaviors That Should be Present at 6 Months
    Comprehension
        Consistent orienting to sound
    Production
        Productive vocalization continues or increases
        Syllable repetition ("ba-ba-ba")
        Duration of cooing, singing, and babbling 2–3 seconds
        Variable intonation, during both crying and cooing
        Voiced-voiceless contrast: /p/ vs /b/
        Discrete tongue movements: /d/n/d/

Behaviors That Should be Present at 12 Months
    Production
        Produces "ma-ma" or "da-da," or pet name referentially; low frequency and intelligibility; imitates speech sounds.
    Comprehension
        Understands his name or name of present familiar person
Responsive to gestured requests to attend to objects
    Use of language for communication
        Turn-taking vocalizations in communication games such as "peek-a-boo" and "pat-a-cake"

Behaviors That Should be Present at 18 Months
    Comprehension
        Understands single words and names for familiar people and objects within visual field
    Production
        Few intelligible words
        Words frequently note familiar people and objects
        Frequency of vocalization increasing
    Use of language for communication
        Requests
        Comments
        Rejects with motor and vocal or just vocal behavior
        "Hi" and "bye" with gesture or vocal behavior

Behaviors That Should be Present at 24 Months
  Comprehension
    Understands at least two words in an utterance, such as "throw ball," indicating action-object relation
    Understands action verbs and reference to absent objects
  Production
    Vocabulary increase to 20 words minimum
    Two-word utterances
  Use of language for communication
    Requests, names, locations, "what's that?"
    Uses words for multiple functions
    Initiates topics in conversation following a pause

Adapted from Miller (1982).

short of that represents a language and communication deficit. It is important to promote as much language learning as possible to make sure that children are able to use language and communication skills that keep pace with their advancing intellectual skills.

PARENTS' AND SIBLINGS' ROLES IN FOSTERING LANGUAGE AND COMMUNICATION DEVELOPMENT

There are essentially six strategies that teachers and family members can use to enhance language and communication development. These six devices are derived from research data on language development and experience in fostering communication in children who have Down syndrome. These techniques are directed toward providing opportunity for reciprocal interaction. They recognize that communication involves each person taking the two primary roles of speaker and listener. Each person must be both expressive and responsive. Essentially, we are trying to do two things: to increase the children's ability to express themselves and to increase the ability to respond through language.

1. Family members and others should be responsive to child-initiated communicative attempts. This means that as the child initiates a communicative gesture, either verbally or nonverbally, it should be responded to immediately and with seriousness. This level of responsiveness should increase the likelihood of such attempts being made again.

2. Through the first 4 years of life, speech should be directed toward immediate, ongoing events, as they relate to words the child knows, as in describing and commenting on the child's activities. Care should be taken to maintain joint attention to these objects and events while talking about them. Essentially, this means that while playing and interacting with the child there should be comments about surrounding objects and events, particularly those for which the child knows the names. Speech should be directed to the child when the child is paying attention, so it isn't just a stream of verbalizations that do not orient the child to what is being talked about. The first step in this process is to get the child's attention, either through saying his or her name or tapping on the objects to be mentioned. Such attentional devices are imperative so that the child can link the verbalization of the word with the object itself.

3. Children should be expected to comprehend more than they are able to say. This doesn't mean that adults should talk in very complex sentences to children. By expecting greater comprehension, we allow children to use what they know about the world to solve verbal problems.

4. Children should be part of routine activities and conversational games, such as ''pat-a-cake'' and ''peek-a-boo.'' These routines provide consistently recurring situations, allowing children to learn turn-taking and reciprocal relationships, which are the foundations of conversational skills. The games also provide circumstances in which the children's expectations are consistently met. Furthermore, these activities combine words and actions in a consistent exchange.

5. When children have acquired a variety of individual words, teachers and family members should repeat the utterances, expanding them by one or two words, particularly when children are imitating an adult utterance that was just said to them. These imitations and opportunities for expansions will be helpful in drawing the attention to multiword utterances and the way in which they are formed in the particular language.

6. It should be recognized that communication skills are the family's responsibility as well as the responsibility of the service system, that is, the school or the speech language pathologist. Communication must be fostered in the children's activities *throughout* their daily routine.

The goal of these six activities is to promote an increased focus on language and communication in everyday life, not to create therapists or teachers out of family members. Using the basic principles discussed in this chapter, it is possible to become more effective in everyday communicative skills without having to set aside a special time or changing the role from parent, or brother, or sister. As more is learned about the language and communication characteristics of children with Down syndrome, more will be understood about the nature of brain and language relationships as well as the conditions under which language can be optimally promoted in this population.

Whoever provides daily care for a child has the greatest opportunity to help that child learn language. My grandmother was at one time a caretaker of children, so, in conclusion, I give you the advice my grandmother gave me on how to converse with them (Miller, 1981).

1. *Listen.* Focus on what the child means by what he or she says so that your responses will show shared focus.

2. *Be patient.* Do not overpower the child with requests or actions. Allow the child space and time to perform. Do not be afraid of pauses.

3. *Follow the child's lead.* Maintain the child's focus (topic, meaning) with responses, comments, and questions and add new information where appropriate. Maintain the child's pace, do not rush on to the next activity.

4. *Value the child.* Recognize the child's comments as important and worth undivided attention.

5. *Learn to think like a child.* Consider the child's perspective at different levels of cognitive development and his or her awareness of varying perspectives of actions, space, and time.

REFERENCES

Miller, J.F. (1981). *Assessing language production in children: Experimental procedures.* Austin, TX: Pro-Ed.

Miller, J.F. (1982). Early Language Intervention: When and how. In M. Lewis & L. Taft (Eds.), Developmental disabilities in the preschool child, early identification, assessment, and intervention strategies, pp. 333–349. Chicago, IL: Spectrum.

Miller, J.F. (1987). Language and communication characteristics of children with Down syndrome. In S. Pueschel, C. Tingey, J. Rynders, A. Crocker, & D. Crutecher (Eds.), *New perspectives on Down syndrome* (pp. 233–262). Baltimore: Brookes.

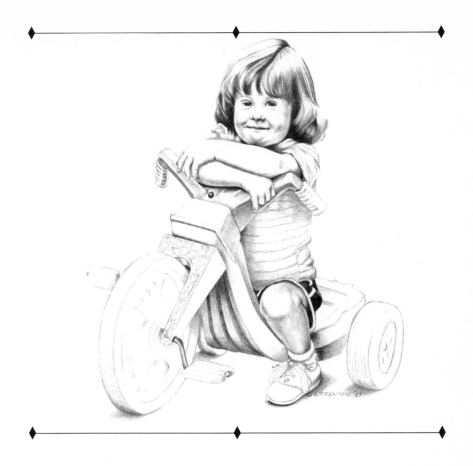

CHAPTER NINE

EARLY INTERVENTION FOR INFANTS AND PRESCHOOLERS WITH DOWN SYNDROME: A REVIEW OF BEST PRACTICES AND EFFECTIVENESS DATA

GLENDON CASTO

◆

Looking at the history of intervention programs for infants and young children with Down syndrome, it becomes apparent that until the 1960s, placement in institutions was the recommended intervention. Indeed, at some institutions, placement of infants with Down syndrome actually increased during the 1950s (Centerwall & Centerwall, 1960).

During the 1960s, more parents began keeping their infants in the home, and home intervention programs began to proliferate. The impetus for these programs was based partly on findings from studies by Centerwall and Centerwall (1960) and Shipe and Shotwell (1965) that infants who spent their early years in their parents' home showed a permanent advantage over children placed in institutions at birth. Early home intervention programs were typically called *infant stimulation programs* and consisted of various types of visual, auditory, and tactile stimulation, movement activities, and maternal handling and affection (Brinkworth, 1973).

In the early 1970s, the Handicapped Children's Early Education program began funding early intervention demonstration programs, and in 1975, a model demonstration program for infants and young children with Down syndrome conducted by the University of Washington was validated for nationwide dissemination by the Joint Dissemination Review Panel (JDRP) of the U.S. Office of Education.

This demonstration program was designed to increase the rate of sensory, vocal, and motor development, and also, since older preschoolers were involved, to increase the rate of preacademic and social performance. A further objective was to involve parents in the intervention program as full participants. The overall goal of the project was to prepare infants and young children with Down syndrome to enter education programs in the public schools.

The home-based programs included an infant learning class that met once a week. In this class, one or both parents received 30 minutes of individualized instruction in sensory-motor development and were then expected to work with their child at home the rest of the week. The bulk of the intervention was delivered at home by the parent.

In the center-based program, the preschool classes met for 2 hours four times per week. Each class consisted of approximately 10 preschoolers, a head teacher, and an assistant teacher. The mothers of the children worked in the classroom one day per week. The interventions were primarily delivered in the center-based setting.

Other JDRP projects intervened with infants and young children with Down syndrome in home-based projects (Casto, 1979), center-based

The work discussed in this chapter was carried out in part with funds from the U.S. Department of Education (Contracts 300-82-0367 and 300-85-0173) to the Early Intervention Research Institute at Utah State University.

projects (Karnes, 1970), and home- and center-based combinations (Fredericks & Moore, 1978). These projects involved parents extensively and utilized project-developed curricula.

The early intervention paradigm utilized with infants and young children with Down syndrome, which represents current best practices, is exemplified by the model program being conducted by the Association for Children with Down Syndrome (ACDS) in Bellmore, NY. This program currently provides services for 120 preschoolers with Down syndrome.

The ACDS preschool program consists of several programs directed at various developmental levels. The infant program is for parents and children from birth to approximately 14 months of age, while the toddler and preschool program is directed at children from 14 months to 5 years of age. At age 5, children are referred to their local public school district's Committee on Special Education for appropriate educational placement.

The philosophy of the entire early intervention program is based on a Piagetian model of development. It is believed that children with Down syndrome follow the same sequence of development as children without Down syndrome and can show gains in developmental skills. Developmental differences between children with and without Down syndrome generally exist with regard to the rate of growth, which is influenced by the level of mental retardation and the home and school environment. The majority of children enter the infant program shortly after birth (approximately 2 months of age). It is at this time that families are introduced to a transdisciplinary team of specialists. A transdisciplinary team differs from other teams in one important dimension. Team members share their expertise freely with one another, and there is considerable interchange among members so that the final program developed for each child represents the best collective thinking of the group. In a transdisciplinary setting, no one discipline predominates. The parents and their infants come to school twice a week, and a special educator who is the primary facilitator sees them each time. The parents meet with the teacher and with other members of the transdisciplinary team who have played major roles in defining the child's individual objectives and goals.

The toddler and preschool programs are held at the school five mornings each week. Children are transported via bus or by their parents to the school. The day at ACDS begins with an individualized sensory program designed by all team members to awaken the children's senses and prepare them for the intensive learning time that is ahead of them that morning. Often, in the toddler programs (ages 1–3), the children have a snack time following sensory stimulation. Children then spend time working on individual skills selected from their Individualized Educational Program. For each child, a unique task box is used. This plastic box has a checklist of daily skills and toys or other objects needed in training that child. As a result, teachers, teacher aides, and volunteers can all easily work with the child in the same way. In all areas of development, each task objective is defined by the team and evaluated by the team.

Task periods are often followed by circle or large group activities. Freeplay time in the classroom is also provided for the children. Outdoor activities are also planned. An adaptive playground is available to meet the children's needs. Children bring lunch daily and also participate in cooking.

A unique feature of the ACDS program is its extensive use of community volunteers. These volunteers are first trained in intervention procedures and then assigned to specific classrooms.

The ACDS program is highly individualized and is based on a variety of curricula. There is a high degree of parent involvement, and parents are unanimously supportive of the program.

Other programs for preschoolers with Down syndrome also serve infants and young children with a variety of other handicapping conditions. In these cases, the programs are also highly individualized, and the curricula utilized are chosen in an eclectic fashion based on the needs of the children served. Most programs emphasize the areas of gross and fine motor skills, language skills, and self-help skills.

There are also programs that mainstream preschoolers with Down syndrome into nursery school and day care settings. It is expected that these types of programs will increase in the future. Both the Social Integration Project (Rule et al., 1985) and the Multi-Agency Project for Preschoolers have mainstreamed preschoolers with Down syndrome.

EVALUATION OF PROGRAM EFFECTIVENESS

Considerable attention has been paid to the evaluation of early intervention for infants and preschoolers with Down syndrome. Although many reviewers of the primary research literature have concluded that early intervention is effective for this population, there is little objective evidence available.

The fact that the efficacy data are so scarce led researchers at the Early Intervention Research Institute at Utah State University to attempt to collect all efficacy studies on Down syndrome as part of a larger integrative review of early intervention efficacy research. Integrative review procedures were used to summarize the data from 16 studies that had been found and that had measurable outcomes and could be coded. The coding system covered the following areas.

1. Introduction (five items, including study identification number, year, and source)

2. A description of the subjects included in the research (20 items, including demographic variables on both infant and family)
3. The type of intervention used (37 items, including type of intervention, the setting, child-intervenor ratio, etc.)
4. The type and quality of research design employed, including presence of various threats to validity and whether data collectors were "blind" (17 items)
5. The type of outcome measured and the procedures used (12 items)
6. The conclusions reached by the study, including the magnitude of the standardized mean difference effect size, the source of that information, and the conclusions of the author (seven items).

For each of the 98 items coded for each study, conventions or coding guidelines were written. For example, intervention setting was coded as follows: 1, intervention is delivered only in home setting, including foster home; 2, intervention is delivered only in nonresidential center-based settings (including Head Start, public school, day care, university, and state social services agencies); 3, intervention delivered in any residential institution, hospital, etc; 4, outpatient services delivered in a doctor's office, clinic, or other center (this includes children who attend a center coded as 2), but only for speech or physical therapy, and who do not participate in a total educational program; 5, other.

The magnitude of the effect attributed to each intervention was estimated using a standard mean difference effect size, defined as ($X_E - X_C$) ÷ SD (Glass, McGaw, & Smith, 1981). This "effect size" measure is essentially the difference between experimental (X_E) and control groups (X_C) measured in standard deviations (SD). This measure has been widely used in recent years to describe the impact of educational programs (Cohen, 1977; Glass, 1976; 1978; Horst, Tallmadge, & Wood, 1975).

It is important to note that one study could yield multiple effect sizes. For example, a study that compared an experimental group with a control group on cognitive and language functioning immediately at the conclusion of an intervention program would yield two effect sizes, one for IQ and one for language.

The meta-analysis of the efficacy literature on children with Down syndrome yielded 43 standardized mean difference effect sizes. The effect sizes included in the analysis came from studies conducted from 1964 to 1984, but mostly since 1970. These studies were reported mostly in medical and psychological journals; but some came from educational journals, books, ERIC documents, government reports, and dissertations. Not surprisingly, the most frequently measured outcome was some type of developmental measure, including motor, IQ, social-emotional, language,and adaptive measures.

DESCRIPTION OF THE INTERVENTIONS

Other than a regimen advocated by Brinksworth (1973, 1975) that included diet, exercise, and socialization activities, most interventions were geared across all developmental domains and featured interventions delivered by professionals, para-professionals, and parents. The reported interventions ranged from a total of 15 hours (Wolf & McAlonie, 1977) to 429 hours (Hayden & Dmietriev, 1975).

Table 9-1 presents an overview of the 16 studies with certain descriptive information and the effect sizes for each study.

RESULTS

The overall results indicate that early intervention programs produce modest developmental gains in infants and young children with Down syndrome. Table 9-2 reports these data.

Further analyses were done to document the effects of variables seen as being important by other reviewers (White, Bush, & Casto, 1985–1986). Their analyses are reported next.

Parental Involvement

Previous reviewers had concluded that intensive parent involvement is associated with intervention effectiveness. Table 9-3 presents the results for Down syndrome. The results indicate that programs that involve parents extensively demonstrate slight advantages (0.10 SD). These findings are not in agreement with the findings from a larger meta-analysis (Casto & Lewis, 1984), which found no differences between programs with extensive parental involvement and programs with little or no involvement.

One study on Down syndrome (Bidder, Bryant, & Gray, 1975) attempted comparisons among different levels of parental involvement and found significant differences favoring the more intensively involved group. However, two qualifications exist with regard to the study. First, the sample sizes were very small (eight experimental subjects and eight control), and second, the Griffiths Developmental Scale was the only outcome measure utilized.

When data from all early intervention studies with children who have Down syndrome are considered with the Bidder et al. (1975) results, there appears to be little difference among programs with various levels of parental involvement.

Parent involvement has always been an important component of early intervention programs. Some intervenors have even insisted that parents

Author/Year	Number of Subjects	Mean Effect Size*	Subject Information	Measures	Program Duration	Type of Stimulation
Aroson & Fallstrom, 1977	6	0.48	8 Experimental 8 Control	Griffiths Griffiths	18 mos. 36 hrs.	All developmental areas All developmental areas
Bidder et al., 1975	1	1.10	8 Experimental 8 Control	Griffiths Griffiths	26 wks. 91 hrs.	Parent training Parent training
Brinkworth, 1973	2	0.22	6 Experimental 12 Control	Griffiths Griffiths	6 mos. 24 hrs.	Diet, exercise, socialization
Brinkworth, 1975	2	1.15	234 Down Syndrome	Griffiths	Not given	Diet, socialization, exercise
Clunies-Ross, 1979	1	1.30	36 Down Syndrome	Developmental profile	Not given	All developmental areas
Connolly et al., 1980	3	0.81	30 Experimental 53 Comparison	S-Binet Vineland	3 yrs. 150 hrs.	Developmental areas Parent training
Drash & Stolberg, 1978	1	0.50	3 Experimental	Cattell	11–35 mos.	Parent training
Ford, 1978	1	1.60	5 Center-based	DDST	31 wks.	Parent training
Haydon & Dimitriev, 1975	3	0.50	8 Experimental	PPVT DDST	62 hrs. 39 wks.	All developmental areas
Hansen, 1978	4	1.51	15 Home-based 10 Experimental	Bayley Bayley	429 hrs. 24 mos.	All developmental areas All developmental areas
Harris, 1981	4	-0.01	10 Control	Peabody Motor	9 wks.	Neurodevelopmental therapy
Mitchell et al., 1981	2	-0.75	14 Experimental	Bayley	16 hrs. 129 wks.	All developmental areas
Piper & Pless, 1980	1	-0.16	21 Experimental 16 Control	Griffiths Griffiths	26 wks. 102 hrs.	Parent training All developmental areas
Shipe & Shotwell, 1965	6	0.26	25 Home-reared 17 Institution	Kuhlmann–Binet Vineland	Not given Not given	Environmental: Home versus institution
Wolf & McAlonie, 1977	2	1.43	8 Center-based	Receptive/Expressive Language	20 wks. 15 hrs.	Receptive & expressive language

*Difference between control group and experimental group measured in standard deviations.

Table 9-2.
Average Effect Size for Down Syndrome Early Intervention Efficacy Studies

	ES	S_{es}	N_{es}
All studies	0.47	0.80	44

Key: ES, mean effect size;
  S_{es}, standard error of the mean for ES;
  N_{es}, number of ESs on which a calculation is based.

be involved intensively. These results suggest that parents should be given more involvement options and then each parent should choose the type and intensity of involvement he or she finds appropriate and meaningful.

Age at Start

The second most frequent conclusion had been that age at start is related to intervention effectiveness (earlier is better). However, the results of the analysis of data about Down syndrome suggest that age at start is not related to intervention effectiveness, a finding in agreement with the Casto and Mastropieri (1986) results. Although one study did find differences favoring younger intervention ages (Brinkworth, 1975), it was a follow-up study with no control group comparisons.

Clearly, both the age at which intervention should start and the degree to which parents should be involved in intervention programs are questions requiring further research with preschoolers with Down syndrome. Other critical research areas include which program components are most useful and comparing home- and center-based options. While continuing to intervene as early as possible, we should seek definitive answers through more tightly controlled research studies.

Table 9-3.
Average Effect Size for Different Levels of Parental Involvement in Intervention

	ES	S_{es}	N_{es}
Extensive involvement	0.50	1.03	21
Little or no involvement	0.40	0.51	18

See Table 9-2 for abbreviations.

CONCLUSION

Although exemplary programs for preschoolers with Down syndrome continue to proliferate, it is surprising, considering the widespread interest in early intervention, that so little efficacy research with infants and young children with Down syndrome has been done. It is also disconcerting to note the generally poor quality of the research done to date. One of the best ways, certainly, to investigate efficacy questions would be a true experimental design so that the critical variable may be actively controlled in the experiment. The use of true experimental designs in research with preschoolers with Down syndrome should be more widely encouraged. There should also be more emphasis on qualitative single-case research with infants and young children with Down syndrome. Tingey (1987), for example, has discovered some significant facts regarding the role of parents in the language development of preschoolers with Down syndrome by studying triplets, of whom one has Down syndrome. More attention should also be paid to other intervention components, including the utilization of procedures to ensure that the treatment program was actively implemented as planned and the use of "blind" examiners.

REFERENCES

Bidder, R.T., Bryant, G., & Gray, O.P. (1975). Benefits of Down's syndrome children through training their mothers. *Archives of Disease in Childhood, 50*, 383–386.

Brinkworth, R. (1973). The unfinished child: Effects of early home training on the mongol infant. In A.D. Clarke & A.M. Clarke (Eds.), *Mental retardation and behavioral research.* London: Churchill-Livingston.

Brinkworth, R. (1975). The unfinished child: Early treatment and training for the infant with Down's syndrome. *Royal Society of Health Journal.*

Casto, G. (Ed.). (1979). *CAMS training manual.* New York: Walker.

Casto, G., & Lewis, A. (1984). Parent involvement in infant and preschool programs. *Journal of the Division for Early Childhood, 9*, 49–56.

Casto, G., & Mastropieri, M.A. (1986). The efficacy of early intervention programs for handicapped children: A meta-analysis. *Exceptional Children, 52*, 417–424.

Centerwall, S.A., & Centerwall, W.R. (1960). A study of children with mongolism reared in the home compared to those reared away. *Pediatrics, --*, 678–684.

Cohen, J. (1977). *Statistical power analysis for the behavioral sciences.* New York: Academic Press.

Fredericks, H.D., & Moore, W.G. (1978). *Data-based classroom for preschool handicapped children: Teaching Research Infant and Child Center.* Unpublished program evaluation report submitted to the Joint Dissemination Review Panel, Washington, DC.

Glass, G.V. (1976). Primary, secondary, and meta-analysis of research. *Educational Researcher, 5*, 3–8.

Glass, G.V. (1978). Reply to Mansfield and Bussey. *Educational Researcher, 7,* 3.

Glass, G.V., McGaw, B., & Smith, M.L. (1981). *Integrating research findings: Meta-analysis in social research.* Beverly Hills: Sage.

Hayden, A.H., & Dmietriev, V. (1975). The multidisciplinary preschool program for Down's syndrome children at the University of Washington model preschool center. In B.Z. Freidlander, G.M. Sterritt, & G.E. Kirk (Eds.), *Exceptional infant, Vol 3: Assessment and intervention.* New York: Brunner/Mazel.

Horst, D.P., Tallmadge, G.K., & Wood, C.T. (1975). *A practical guide to measuring project impact on student achievement* (No. 1, Stock No. 017-080-01460-2). Washington, DC: U.S. Government Printing Office.

Karnes, M.B. (1970). *Precise early education of children with handicaps (PEECH).* Champaign, IL: Colonel Wolfe Preschool Building.

Rule, S., Killoran, J., Stowitschek, J.J., Innocenti, M., Striefel, S., & Boswell, C. (1985). Training and support for mainstream day care staff. *Early Child Development and Care, 20,* 99–113.

Shipe, D., & Shotwell, A.M. (1965). Effect of out of home care on mongoloid children: A continuation study. *American Journal of Mental Deficiency, 69,* 649–652.

Tingey, C. (1987). *Language development in triplets, one of whom has Down syndrome.* Unpublished manuscript, Early Intervention Research Institute, Utah State University, Logan, Utah.

White, K.R., Bush, D.W., & Casto, G. (1985–86). Learning from previous reviews of early intervention research. *Journal of Special Education, 19,* 417–428.

Wolf, J.M., & McAlonie, M.L. (1977). A multimodality language program for retarded preschoolers. *Education and Training of the Mentally Retarded, 12,* 127–131.

PART FOUR

EDUCATION AND COMMUNITY ACTIVITIES

For most children kindergarten is the beginning of formal education. This right of passage is a time of celebration for many families, but for families of children with Down syndrome reaching kindergarten age can be a startling experience that brings them face to face with the difficulties caused by the child's developmental delays.

School personnel and parents are challenged to work together to develop a curriculum that will provide an educational experience that is neither too demanding nor passive for the child. Parents continue their role as educational advocates by becoming involved in decisions regarding Individual Education Plans and proper school placements for their children.

By the time most students with Down syndrome are of junior high school age, they have been taught some reading and writing skills. However, these reading and writing skills usually are not adequate for study in high school textbooks, and most of these secondary school level students will experience more success in activity classes rather than in subject matter classes. Classes involving learning through activities and laboratory experiences, not abstract topics, are best suited to the skills of students with Down syndrome. Direct, relevant experiences for secondary school-aged students with Down syndrome are centered largely around preparation for the ''career of life'' through vocational education.

Individuals with Down syndrome need to be prepared not only for the world of work, but also for an interpersonal world requiring social competence. Adults with Down syndrome can participate with other adults in their community during their off-work hours. To interact with people it is important that they learn acceptable ways to manage their own behavior and relate appropriately to others in recreational and social situations.

This final section of this book covers the transition into school, and from school into adult life for people with Down syndrome. Chapter 10 addresses various issues for educators and parents to consider in establishing an optimal elementary school environment for students with Down syndrome. Progression to secondary school is the focus of Chapter 11. At the junior high and high school level vocational education is introduced to prepare these students for adult life. Finally, Chapter 12 describes training techniques to develop personal recreational skills in adults with Down syndrome. Equipped with the necessary vocational and interpersonal skills, adults with Down syndrome can remain active and welcome members of their community.

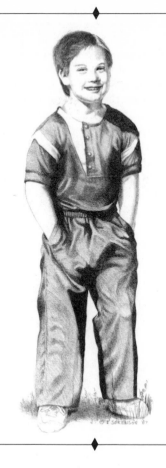

CHAPTER TEN

ELEMENTARY SCHOOL EXPERIENCE

CAROL TINGEY

♦

Learning theorists disagree on how people learn. There are two rather rigidly divided positions. Some theorists see learning as happening only through direct sensorial experience (empiricism or behavioral-associative theory). Others see learning as primarily the result of reason and intuition (rationalism or cognitive-organizational theory). Both positions state that there must be a stimulus in order for learning to happen, but theorists disagree on exactly what that stimulus is or should be and how the learner uses the stimulus. The behavioral-associative theorists claim that learning can be directed only through physical participation in activity. The cognitive-organizational theorists suggest that learning can be directed by supplying stimulus for the learner to ponder (Bower & Hilgard, 1981).

Jean Piaget (1952, 1962; Flavell, 1963), whose studies of children's development span many decades, suggested that learning happens both ways. Piaget saw that early learning, whether in a young child or in an adult coming in contact with something new, is always sensory or experiential learning. According to Piaget, once a topic or skill becomes more familiar to the learner, the learning then happens largely through cognition. As a result, as an individual learns more, he or she is able to learn more quickly and efficiently.

Learning, according to all learning theorists, is also at least partly related to the physiological capabilities of the learner. Some people are physically able to respond, and therefore learn at a much faster rate than others.

LEARNING OF BABIES AND CHILDREN

Although most people who have not studied learning theory are not aware of the theories and the research to support the theories, there is a rather large body of conventional wisdom on how learning can be facilitated for children. Those who provide care for toddlers and young children know that toys and playgrounds are important. When the child reaches "school age," however, toys and playgrounds are seen as for before and after school, and the child is expected to sit in a seat, use crayons and scissors, and learn to read about Dick and Jane. This format for formal education appears to be successful for most children. By the time most children reach the chronological age for school, they have experienced enough toys, play yards, and sensory-motor experiences to be ready to use symbols to represent those experiences. The ability to handle symbols quickly and with agility is necessary in order to follow the instructions in elementary school.

LEARNING OF CHILDREN WITH DOWN SYNDROME

Due largely to delayed development, children with Down syndrome have more difficulty with symbol representation and with language that is not related to the present time or things that can be seen. Children with

Down syndrome need more sensory-motor experiences in order to reach a point at which they can profit from hours of verbal instruction from a teacher. The usual "sit down and learn" is not the most appropriate elementary school experience for children with Down syndrome. (There is some question as to whether it is the *best* way for any early elementary school-aged child to learn, but that is another issue [Michaelis, 1981b].) Not only is the developmental age of the school-aged child with Down syndrome more like that of most preschool children, but even when mental age increases, learning is still facilitated more readily in a doing rather than in a thinking atmosphere. Children with Down syndrome are especially good at learning to do what they see others doing, in apprentice-like fashion.

LOCATION OF ELEMENTARY SCHOOLING

There is no reason that appropriate elementary education cannot be provided for children with Down syndrome in the regular elementary school building (Fredricks, Mushlitz, & DeRoest, 1987; Michaelis, 1981a). Learning-by-doing means only that the day-to-day experience needs to be one in which there is space and time for children to explore and actively try things out. Being an active participant in the learning setting means not only that children have the opportunity to see, touch, feel, and handle concrete objects, but also that children are encouraged and rewarded for physically trying. This requires an instructor who can mix the skills of an early education teacher and an elementary school teacher. It also requires an instructional format that is a cross between planned formal instruction and making the most of opportunities for incidental teaching. Effective teachers for children with Down syndrome must be able to plan activities yet also be able to "go with the flow." These specialized learning opportunities, however, do not need an isolated special school setting. They can be provided in a classroom in a regular elementary school building.

EDUCABLE VERSUS TRAINABLE

There has been discussion during recent years concerning the educational label of school-aged children with Down syndrome (Pueschel, Tingey, Rynders, Chocker, & Crutchen, 1987). Parents and members of advocacy organizations are anxious to have the child receive the "highest" placement in a school setting and therefore campaign for the educable label. The exact cutoff for educable and trainable labels varies from state to state and sometimes within states, but the educable label is always given for a higher measured IQ score and therefore implies a greater ability to learn.

Although labels may be necessary for classification, it is not likely that a mere label will influence children's abilities to learn. A careful evaluation of all of the children's abilities, including daily life skills, is of more practical importance than the degree of mental retardation measured through psychological examination. Sternberg's research concerning intelligence and his descriptions of "intelligent behavior" suggest that the ability to get along with others and to problem solve is perhaps more significant than a score on a standardized test (Sternberg, 1985; Sternberg & Wagner 1986). Elementary school-aged children with Down syndrome frequently show what Sternberg labels as "street-wise" intelligence, (Tingey, 1987a).

Care should always be taken, however, to see that all evaluation measures are given in such a way that children are able to generate the highest IQ rating possible in each psychological examination. A lower than necessary IQ score can cause unrealistically low expectations in those around a child. Children with Down syndrome usually get higher scores on psychological measures that sample more than just language skill. It is important that the child is feeling well the day of the examination and that the examiner has had experience working with children who have Down syndrome. No child performs well when testing situations are not planned adequately. It is especially important that the child with Down syndrome is tested in a comfortable, familiar setting and that the testing procedure is not hurried.

Although the IQ score is frequently used to determine whether the child is labeled educable or trainable, and sometimes the physical placement of the child is made from that label, it is actually not the label but the content of the curriculum and the setting where the training takes place that is important. Elementary school-aged children with Down syndrome profit greatly from contact with other children their own chronological age. If a child's classroom is in the regular school building, and appropriate activities are implemented, the label given to a child may have little significance.

CURRICULUM CONTENT

A major concern should be the content of the curriculum. The regular elementary school curriculum concentrates on learning basic reading, writing, and arithmetic skills in order for children to use these skills in the pursuit of subject matter in high school and beyond. This focus may not be appropriate for a child with Down syndrome. Although there is no reason why the child cannot learn the basic skills, the learning of these skills must be couched in real-life experience rather than the drill of a worksheet. Children with Down syndrome need to learn to read the names of others in the class and the items on a grocery list rather than the sequenced list of words that describe the idealistic life of Dick and Jane. Children with Down syndrome need to learn to tell time and count change rather than to learn the procedures for short division, practiced on sheets of newsprint. Children with Down syndrome need to learn to write their name and address rather than the sentences to practice this week's spelling words.

CAREER EDUCATION

One of the difficulties that all learners experience is learning something in one setting and actually being able to use that learning in another setting. Forward-thinking professionals concerned not only with the years that the child spends in the classroom, but also with the usefulness of those experiences in later life, suggest that even children without learning problems profit more from applied instruction. Certainly this is true for children with learning problems because part of their problem is being able to transfer basic skills to another task (Smith, 1968). If the activities in the school are closely related to the activities of life, children have less difficulty learning to transfer the things learned in school to a real-life time and place. This philosophy is called career education, and it suggests that children be trained not in how to complete worksheets, but in how to deal with the problems that occur in life (Brolin, 1978; Brolin & Elliott, 1984).

The Cincinnati Curriculum for Slow Learners (1964) lists 13 persisting life problems, including the needs to keep healthy, communicate with others, and to use leisure time wisely. Most children are expected, somehow, to learn these things incidently while they are learning spelling words, completing worksheets, and memorizing the multiplication tables. Since children with Down syndrome have the right to school experiences that are tailored especially for them, it is possible to look at each child separately and devise individual learning experiences to meet each child's needs. These experiences will be most effective if they are rich in activities that are very similar to the doing activities of daily life. (Later in this chapter the process for development of the Individual Educational Plan [IEP] is discussed.)

READING INSTRUCTION

For years, educators of children with Down syndrome did not consider reading to be something that could be achieved by these children. In recent years, it has been shown again and again that this is not true. There may be processes of teaching reading that are more beneficial, however, than the usual learning of the alphabet and sounds for the letters of the alphabet, followed by learning rules for the combination of letters.

Rather than approaching reading in an analytical manner, children with Down syndrome could learn more effectively by approaching reading as a game to label things already familiar to the child. Recognition of the child's name and the names of family members, pets, and friends is a good beginning. Next, the words for the child's favorite foods, activities, restaurants, and television shows can be added. Rather than trying to make the life of Dick and Jane real, it is much more effective to have the child tell a story that is already real. Then the teacher can illustrate that story with actual pictures about things that the child has already experienced and already knows. Learning labels for things that are already familiar is a much more effective way of learning how to decode written symbols. Of course, there is no reason why the child can't use the regular reading series for supplemental reading, if the child is doing well and is interested in the other books.

Most children with Down syndrome need encouragement and opportunity to practice verbal skills. The creating of story books is also an experience that encourages verbal expression. Some of the stories could be about how to wait for, get on, and ride the bus (Michaelis, 1981c) or how to handle the lunch tray or other skills that are needed in daily life (Michaelis, 1981d). It can also be beneficial to have children act out their own or other children's stories. Although the adults may see the plot of the story as thin, children will find it fascinating to represent the situation as they see it.

WRITING

The fine motor skill necessary for holding a pencil is something that children develop after they have had experience with large motor activities. Fluency in fine motor skill is frequently difficult for the child with Down syndrome. Continual practice of any difficult skill is not as effective as ample practice performing prerequisite skills that are just below the difficult skill on the developmental scale. This means first the child needs fluency in holding and using larger objects such as combs, toothbrushes, silverware, buttons, and handles. All children differ in their fine motor skills, and some children with Down syndrome, even after appropriate preparation and practice, may still have difficulty writing clearly. For these children, alternate means of writing could be considered, such as typewriting or computer keyboarding. All children, however, should be taught to write their own name, even if the process is tedious and time-consuming and the result not easy to decipher. It is easy for others to treat someone who cannot write their name as a nonperson. Performing the social art of signing a paper is more important than the legibility of the signature. There is a rather large number of very successful people who have signatures that can hardly be read. (Maybe that is why business letters have the typed name below the signature.)

ARITHMETIC

Numbers are labels to represent things that can be classified into groups that are similar. It is necessary for the child to first see how things are similar. Then the child can learn to describe the number of similar things that are present in a particular situation. For children with Down syndrome, the ability to perform addition, subtraction, multiplication, and division on abstract numbers is not nearly as important as the ability to use one-to-one correspondence to figure out how many chairs, cups, plates, or other objects are needed for a group. Unless the child is counting real things, the math functions are meaningless.

Numbers are also parts of addresses and telephone numbers. In these situations, the number may not represent an ordinal sequence, but simply a label. Children with Down syndrome need to know their own address and telephone number, even if they learn them by continual practice and drill. It is also possible for children to learn the telephone numbers of other children in the class and of grandparents and other relatives. A class phone book may be a helpful way of learning the concept with practical application. (Be sure to have permission from the family before listing anyone in the special phone book.) Appropriate telephone manners must also be discussed, demonstrated, and practiced.

Telling time is an important part of participating in the mainstream of life in the United States. Appointments, dates, schedules, and meals all happen at certain times. Knowing how to read the clock is part of being in the right place at the right time, ready for the appropriate activity. The digital clock is easier to read, but it has some disadvantages because we usually express time not as, for instance, 2:45, but as a quarter to three. Children need to learn to read both regular and digital clocks. Having a rather large clock of each kind side by side in the classroom and commenting on the time as activities are changed is a good way to help the child associate routine activity with time. Children with Down syndrome are usually happy to participate in regular routines if they know when the activity is to happen. They can prepare themselves for the change of activity better if they learn to keep track of time for themselves.

The use of money is an important skill that takes experience to master. Rather than using the usual worksheets, the child needs the opportunity to purchase things and to handle and count real bills and coins. Although it may seem like a nuisance to both parents and teachers, having the child bring lunch or snack money daily and having children take turns being cashier and giving receipts is an effective way to understand both the meaning and practical use of money.

LANGUAGE LEARNING

One of the significant problems of children and adults with Down syndrome is the difficulties in using language (see Chapter 8). An important reason for special education placement is that the number of children in the class is smaller, and therefore each child has more opportunity to talk. It is important that the classroom atmosphere encourages children to talk and adults and other children to listen. Teachers of elementary school-aged children with Down syndrome can facilitate these activities with daily show-and-tell activities. Other ways to encourage language practice include role playing and taking turns being "teacher." Although receptive language may be facilitated while the child is sitting quietly in the seat, improvement in expressive language can only happen when the child is talking.

HEALTH AND DIET

One of the goals of education for any child is the development of independent adult skills. Early learning concerning rest, proper diet, and other health needs is important for children with Down syndrome. Dietary habits established in the elementary school years are the basis for life-long eating patterns. As any adult knows, maintaining a healthy weight is more difficult as we get older. Short stature and slow movement patterns combined with difficulties in thyroid function contribute to a tendency toward weight problems for many adults with Down syndrome. Learning to snack on fresh fruits and vegetables may be difficult for some children because oral motor problems may make softer foods "feel" better (see Chapter 7), but such learning can facilitate lifelong health. If the children peel and slice together, the treat is more fun because they share in the preparation. (This activity is also an ideal time for natural language practice.) Yogurt flavored with spices can make a low-calorie dip. One special education teacher planned with the children all week for a Friday afternoon cooking session (usually using an electric frying pan brought from home). Each child participated by measuring, counting spoonfuls, stirring, or whatever else was appropriate for that child.

Keeping track of going-to-bed and getting-up times can help children learn that efficient activities for the day depend on ample rest at night. Exercise is also extremely important to children with Down syndrome.

A teacher-lead fast walk around the playground in the middle of the day is beneficial to all. It is also important to have some movement activities as part of the classroom activity. With the help of a physical or occupational therapist, movements particularly helpful for each child can be designed. Developmental movement activities can also be arranged as a circuit in which the child performs one activity after another or is assigned to work on some movement pattern that is particularly needed (Tingey-Michaelis, 1983a). When motor activities are being planned, it is important to look at the quality of the movement or the way the child moves, not just whether the activity takes place (see Chapter 7).

GROOMING AND APPEARANCE

Vital to the acceptance of others is appearance. No one wants to associate with a person who has a runny nose and untied shoes (Michaelis, 1972, 1979a, 1979b, 1979c; Tingey, 1987b). Although grooming and appearance usually begin at home when the child participates in the self-care skills of early childhood, continued training is necessary. Routines that stress cleanliness and neatness in school are important. One teacher implemented a "Joe Cool" program in which children checked themselves in a full-length mirror adjacent to a full-sized cartoon figure of a "gentleman" with combed hair, clean face, shirttail tucked in, shoes tied, and a smile on his face (Tingey, 1987b). It is not possible for people to look neat all day, unless they learn to check in the mirror after recess and to wipe their face with a napkin during lunch (Michaelis, 1979d).

Looking through catalogues and discussing appropriate clothes for school and other occasions as well as a field trip to the local mall can help young children with Down syndrome develop skills in knowing what is appropriate for various occasions. Not only must one be clean, but wearing a party dress to school is just as unacceptable as not washing one's face. One therapist suggests that children with Down syndrome might want to leave on their jackets because they like the feel of the coat against their skin, but wearing a warm jacket in the spring or no coat on a cold day sets the child apart from others.

Although clean hair and skin originate at home, discussion about cleanliness and practice performing the necessary skills in the classroom are also appropriate. Children with Down syndrome usually have dry skin, and it may be helpful to have lotion available at school. One first-grade teacher has each child bring a box of tissue in the fall so there is a supply for the year. It might be wise also for children to bring bottles of lotion to put on their hands after washing. Dry, cracked skin is most unattractive, and learning to take care of the problem regularly is important.

MOBILITY AND SAFETY

Living in the mainstream means being able to walk around the neighborhood and community independently. Although many children with Down syndrome will live too far from the school they attend to walk to school, if they live close enough, the walk to and from the school could be as significant as the activities in the classroom. Parents and teachers should practice with the child to find the most efficient route and to measure the amount of time necessary for the child to walk to and from the school. That way parents and teachers know when to expect the child to arrive.

Children who must travel to and from school on a bus should learn to wait for the bus independently and to board the bus without assistance both at home and at school. Obviously, this means that someone is ''shadowing'' the child so there is no possibility for danger, but the child will still feel responsible for being in the right place at the right time. The child must learn to attend to the danger of traffic, which will always be close by any bus stop. This means that getting ready for the bus, waiting for the bus, and getting on the bus at the end of the school day are not hurried but are practiced as part of the curriculum. Learning proper behavior on the bus is also an important part of the elementary school curriculum. Field trips are helpful partly because of the activity, but also because the child needs to have appropriate bus behavior complimented by the teacher while the activity is taking place.

Mobility can also be enhanced through classroom shopping trips to the local grocery store for health snacks. Waiting for lights and crossing the street properly are skills that can be developed during walking trips around the school neighborhood. It may be possible to get invitations to come and see things that the neighbors have, such as puppies, goldfish, flowers, quilts, or the construction of an addition to a house. Conversation during the walk helps facilitate language skills. Children with Down syndrome frequently have difficulty asking for assistance. Asking for directions can be programmed into the walking trip.

Also part of the mobility experience is participation in activities that can be done in spare time just for fun. These can be movement games and activities located in the community. Field trips to parks close to children's homes can help the children develop social skills to use with other children. They can also help children become comfortable enough with the play area that they can learn to participate with minimal supervision. In addition to the physical space for recreation, the elementary school-aged child with Down syndrome needs to learn to handle the equipment of the activity. Since learning by doing is effective, the child can learn to participate in anything from gymnastics and swimming to golf and skiing, depending on the opportunity to watch and participate with others.

CLASSROOM DUTIES

Although most of us remember erasing chalkboards and emptying the trash in the school classroom, we seldom appreciate the things that we learned from helping the teacher. For the elementary school-aged child with Down syndrome, cooperation and participation in classroom duties have more potential for education than sit-and-learn activities of most regular classrooms. Being able to take care of plants or pets helps instill understanding of the need for consistent care for living things. Playground, hall, or bus monitoring responsibilities encourage development of responsibility in public situations. Care of play equipment or classroom materials helps children understand how to take care of their own things as well as items that might be used later in the work setting. Although it may seem counterproductive, it can be valuable for the teacher to create enough jobs for each child to always have a job assignment. The assignments can be rotated so that children have the opportunity to participate in a variety of activities. If the assignments are posted, the children can learn to recognize and complete their jobs without being reminded.

INDIVIDUAL EDUCATIONAL PROGRAMS

Perhaps the most significant part of public education for elementary school-aged children with Down syndrome is the requirement of PL 94-142 that each child have an Individual Educational Program [IEP] (Michaelis, 1980; Weisenfeld, 1986). This means that education for children with Down syndrome should not come "off the rack," and they should not have to be assigned to whatever other children are doing. Each child with Down syndrome has the right to educational experiences that are particularly designed for his or her own needs. Not only does the child have the right to special services, but those special services should be designed after this individual child's strengths and weaknesses have been measured. If the educational program is implemented as designed, each child with Down syndrome would have his or her own unique set of school goals and school experiences. Some of these experiences might be similar to other children with Down syndrome or other children in the classroom, but that would not necessarily be true.

The process for the development of the IEP varies slightly depending on where the child lives, and procedures and forms will be different, but there are some general requirements that must be met. First, the situation must be discussed with the parents and permission must be given for the child to be assessed. For so many years it was thought that all children with Down syndrome were alike, and it was assumed that everyone already knew what a child with Down syndrome needed. This is a fallacy. Parents should insist on a complete developmental evaluation, and school personnel should design a battery that includes individual evaluation of all developmental domains as well as instruments to assess concerns that the parents may have about their child. This evaluation should be made by people who have specific training in speech and language, motor development, psychology, social work, medicine, as well as an educational assessment. The evaluators should also have had ample experience working with children who have Down syndrome.

When the assessment is completed and reports are written, the parents and educational personnel meet to determine which potential goals are a priority for the child. When it has been determined exactly what the child is ready to learn and what learning experiences will facilitate that learning, it is time to begin to decide where the child can receive that training most effectively. The location of the educational experience is not nearly as important as the content of the program. The law, however, states clearly that the child should be educated in the school to which the child would ordinarily go unless the educational needs (as determined by the assessment and the goal setting process) cannot be met in that school (Federal Register, 1977).

The IEP is intended to be a working plan that is changed as the parents or the educators see that a change is necessary. Although there is to be at least one meeting a year, more can be scheduled. One of the most efficient ways to update the IEP is to have regular home-to-school and school-to-home communication. A notebook sent back and forth with the child is one of the most efficient ways to accomplish continual, efficient communication. The teacher or other educational worker writes in the notebook things that the child has done at school and parents respond with things that have occurred at home. Regular communication can make it possible to be clear concerning how things are happening and make it unnecessary for parents or teachers to be surprised at formal meeting times (Michaelis, 1980a).

MAINSTREAM EDUCATION

Since children with Down syndrome learn effectively from observation and imitation of others, there is a distinct advantage in having other children around who are performing desirable skills. If educational experiences need to be altered in order to meet practical life goals, especially for older elementary school-aged children, it may be possible to have contact with other children on the playground and in the lunchroom. If this kind of contact is to be used most effectively, then it is important that the child is not just on the playground or in the lunchroom, but that appropriate supervision or training is given in order for the child to be able to use the opportunities effectively. Some teachers have found that a "special playmate" can be selected and trained to help the child with Down syndrome into the regular social and play circles. The selection, training, reinforcement, and supervision of the special playmate become the responsibility of the special education personnel serving the child.

Children with Down syndrome frequently have sisters and brothers close in age who are also attending elementary school. It is important to consider their needs too (Michaelis, 1979a, 1980a, 1981a, 1981e). Although it may seem expedient from the school's point of view to have siblings serve as special playmates, it might be more effective over time to allow other siblings to be free of school responsibility since they may already have many responsibilities for the sibling with Down syndrome at home (Hayden, 1974; Michaelis, 1980a; Michaelis, 1981e) (see Chapter 6).

When kindergarten-aged children with Down syndrome have had ample preschool learning experiences, they can sometimes have their schooling needs met in a regular kindergarten class. If this is determined to be the best placement, then there must be cooperation between the special education personnel and the kindergarten teacher. Although legally it may be possible to force the kindergarten teacher to take the child, common sense suggests that cooperation is something that must be developed rather than mandated. Suggestions for teachers working together include frequent, brief meetings to discuss needs and the planning and supplementation of special curriculum materials, to be the responsibility of the special education teacher (Michaelis, 1980b).

PREPARING THE OTHER CHILDREN

The words of the song from *South Pacific*, "You've got to be taught to be afraid of people whose eyes are oddly made," have some real implications for educators and parents. If the children in the regular classrooms of the school are not taught to understand and accept the child with Down syndrome, they might notice only the differences in appearance and the slowness and not want to be around the child. Active conversations by adults with the other children in the school can serve a variety of purposes: (a) they can satisfy the other children's curiosity; (b) they can be the springboard for requests for special playmates; and (c) they can help the regular teachers as well as the children understand the child with Down syndrome better. Small group discussion appears to be most productive for interaction. Special educational personnel or parents might attend each class and briefly explain what Down syndrome is medically and what it means to learning and development. Then it is important to allow the children in the class an opportunity to ask questions.

HOMEWORK FOR ELEMENTARY SCHOOL-AGED
CHILDREN WITH DOWN SYNDROME

With careful planning, the school curriculum can be continued in the home. There are ample opportunities for development of self-reliance in getting ready for and getting to school. Instruction in telling time can be continued from the school to the home. Getting up and ready for school on time is an important skill for elementary school-aged children, but it must be cultivated even earlier in order for the child to be able to receive benefit from later vocational training. All of the above activities can be tied to learning to read; so can the assignment of routine household chores. It is important that chores assigned be concrete and specific and not too easy or too difficult for the child to accomplish. The chores must also be consistent with chores given to other children in the family (Tingey-Michaelis, 1983b).

Elementary school-aged children with Down syndrome can be expected to perform such chores as making beds, setting the table, loading the dishwasher, vacuuming the floor, and taking out the garbage (Michaelis, 1981d). They can also walk the dog or even be trained to deliver newspapers with supervision and assistance with collection and on stormy days. Since the connection between learning at home and learning at school is so strong, wise educational personnel will work with parents to share success experiences in both settings. If teachers and parents use the same phrases and routines with the child who has Down syndrome, both will have more success.

PREPARING TO LEAVE ELEMENTARY SCHOOL

For all children, the jump from one class and one teacher to the multiple teachers and activities of middle school or junior high school is a difficult change. For children with Down syndrome, this change is perhaps more difficult; for many children and their parents, entering the teenage years is a time of realization of a more global meaning of the impact of mental retardation. Along with the realization comes the concern that in adulthood the child will likely not be completely independent. Other children are growing into more and more competence and independence in academic skills and in social interaction. They are being invited to group dating activities and finding best friends to share homework and social activities. The child with Down syndrome has been able to keep up with the elementary school structure and activities but now faces moving into a more grown-up school setting without grade level, academic, or social skills. This can be a frightening experience for both the child and the parents.

The fear of the situation can be minimized if there are frequent and early visits to the new setting. Recreational activities sponsored by the middle school or junior high school are usually open to the public. If the child and the family attend the school carnival or the spring festival in the school building for years, the location can become more familiar to the child. Elementary school teachers can take children to daytime games, assemblies, or other activities at the school. If the school is close enough, walking trips should include walking on the sidewalk in front of the middle or junior high school. In the spring of the year, arrangements should be made for the child who is graduating from elementary school to spend part of the school day in the new setting. If the child's teacher is not able to go along, then a parent or the special friend or someone else the child already knows should be there.

Moving into a new school does not change the child's abilities or skills, and care must be taken to continue to expect the child to perform well. It is also important not to suddenly expect the child to have the skills of middle or junior high school students without Down syndrome. From a learning point of view, the last day of elementary school is no different than the first day of middle or junior high school. In fact, if there has been a summer in between and the child has been appropriately busy with nonschool activities, the child might be rusty in some school skills. Parents and educators must not allow the child's age or the location or label of the school to influence expectations. The educational expectation for all children, including those with Down syndrome, should not be what are the other children learning; rather, goals should be based on what an individual child is ready to learn each day.

REFERENCES

Bower, G.H., & Hilgard, E.R. (1981). *Theories of Learning*. Englewood Cliffs, NJ: Prentice-Hall.

Brolin, D. (1978). *Life-centered career education: A competency-based approach*. Reston, VA: The Council for Exceptional Children.

Brolin, D.E., & Elliott, T.R. (1984). Meeting the lifelong career development needs of students with handicaps: A community college model. *Career Development for Exceptional Individuals, 7*, 12–21.

Cincinnati Public Schools. (1964). *The slow learning program in elementary and secondary schools*. (Bulletin No. 119). Cincinnati, OH: Author.

Federal Register. (1977). 42(163).

Flavel, J. (1963). *The developmental psychology of Jean Piaget*. Princeton, NJ: VanNostrand.

Fredericks, B., Mushlitz, J., & DeRoest, C. (1987). Integration of children with Down syndrome at the elementary school level: A pilot study. In S. Pueschel, C. Tingey, J.E. Rynders, A.C. Crocker, & D. Crutcher (Eds.), *New perspectives on Down syndrome* (pp. 179–194). Baltimore, MD: Brookes.

Hayden, V. (1974). The other children. *The Exceptional Parent, 4*(4), 26–29.

Michaelis, C.T. (1972). Why can't Johnnie look nice too? *The Exceptional Parent, 1*(5), 24–27.

Michaelis, C.T. (1979a). The readiness of the child and the school. *The Exceptional Parent, 9*(5), R4–R5.

Michaelis, C.T. (1979b). Why can't Johnnie look nice, too? Revisited. Part 1. *The Exceptional Parent, 9*(2), 11–14.

Michaelis, C.T. (1979c). Why can't Johnnie look nice, too? Revisited. Part 2. *The Exceptional Parent, 9*(3), 9–14.

Michaelis, C.T. (1979d). *Self-care skills.* Long Beach, NJ: Kimbo Educational.

Michaelis, C.T. (1980a). *Home and school partnerships in exceptional education.* Rockville, MD: Aspen System Publishers.

Michaelis, C.T. (1980b). Two teachers, one child. *Early Years, 10*(5), 56–57.

Michaelis, C.T. (1981a). Mainstreaming: A mother's perspective. *Topics in Early Childhood Education, 1*(1), 11–16.

Michaelis, C.T. (1981b). How to create a classroom management system to include a hyperactive child. *Early Years, 12*(3), 33.

Michaelis, C.T. (1981c). *Vocational skills.* Long Branch, NJ: Kimbo Educational.

Michaelis, C.T. (1981d). *Housekeeping tasks.* Long Branch, NJ: Kimbo Educational.

Michaelis, C.T. (1981e). Families make the difference. *Exceptional Parent, 11*(3), 40–48.

Piaget, J. (1952). *The origin of intelligence in children.* New York: International Universities Press.

Piaget, J. (1962). *Play, dreams, and imitation in childhood.* New York: Norton.

Pueschel, S., Tingey, C., Rynders, J.E., Crocker, A.C., & Crutcher, D. (1987). *New perspectives on Down syndrome.* Baltimore, MD: Brookes.

Smith, R.M. (1968). *Clinical teaching methods of instruction for the retarded.* New York, NY: McGraw-Hill.

Sternberg, R.J. (1985). *Beyond IQ: A triarchic theory of human intelligence.* Cambridge, MA: Cambridge University Press.

Sternberg, R.J., & Wagner, R.K. (1986). *Practical intelligence nature and origins of competence in the everyday world.* Cambridge, MA: Cambridge University Press.

Tingey, C. (1987a). Psycho social development in individuals with Down syndrome. In S.M. Pueschel, C. Tingey, J. Rynders, A. Crocker, & D. Crutcher (Eds.), *New perspectives on Down syndrome* (pp. 311–344). Baltimore, MD: Brookes.

Tingey, C. (1987b). Advice on good grooming. *The Exceptional Parent, 17*(3), 10–26.

Tingey-Michaelis, C. (1983a). Make room for movement. *Early Years, 13*(6), 26–29.

Tingey-Michaelis, C. (1983b). Homework vs. school work. *The Exceptional Parent, 13*(4), 36–37.

Weisenfeld, R.B. (1986). The IEPs of Down syndrome children: A content analysis. *Education and Training of the Mentally Retarded, 21*(3), 211–219.

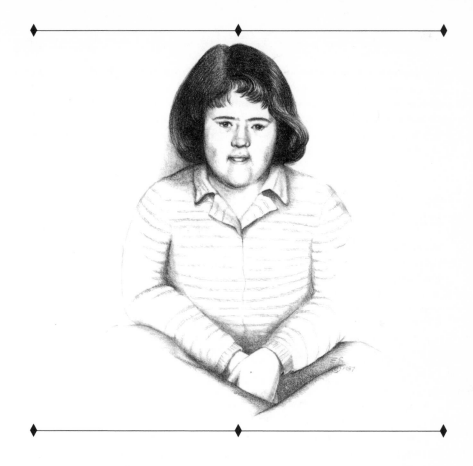

CHAPTER ELEVEN

COMPETITIVE EMPLOYMENT TRAINING AT THE HIGH SCHOOL LEVEL

BUD FREDERICKS

♦

The secondary-school curriculum for students with Down syndrome consists of four major areas, only one of which is vocational. The others are social-sexual skills, practical living skills, and leisure skills. The social-sexual curriculum is vitally important and includes the teaching of relationships and communication skills. It pervades and is an integral part of each of the other curricular components, for within each there are elements of interactions with peers, authority figures, significant others, and the general public. How teenagers and young adults learn to interact with people will largely determine their success with other people, regardless of what other skills they may possess.

Practical living skills include (a) care of one's own body, encompassing personal hygiene, health, and adornment; (b) care of one's living space and possessions, including clothing and the ability to select appropriate clothing; and (c) survival skills, including shopping, cooking, storing of food, mobility around the community, and the entire range of academics, which should be functionally oriented.

The final broad area of curriculum includes leisure skills, which are composed of group or solitary activities and participatory or observational involvement (see Chapter 12).

VOCATIONAL CURRICULUM EMPHASIS

For students with Down syndrome, vocational training time should be increased. At the middle school or junior high school level, approximately 5 or 6 hours a week of such training is ideal. As the student moves through the high school grades, until about age 18, the number of hours should be gradually increased until approximately 10–12 hours a week are devoted to vocational training. Some models of secondary vocational training devote almost 100% of school time to vocational training at ages 18–21.

PREVOCATIONAL TRAINING

The term *prevocational* implies getting ready to work or getting ready to be trained to work. Prevocational training traditionally has been implemented in a number of ways. The most common form of such training has students performing some vocational task such as separating bolts and nuts and then assembling them or sorting other types of materials. The entire school environment should teach work habits through the student's normal interaction with the proffered curriculum. The best training for the world of work is *in* the world of work, and, thus, most prevocational skills can best be taught in the community with a trainer.

However, there are some prevocational skills that can be taught in a classroom in the practical living skills curricular area. These include such activities as locating jobs in the want ads, filling out job applications, and role-playing interviews for jobs.

ASSOCIATED WORK SKILLS

There are other skills that are sometimes included under the term prevocational. These are associated work skills. A list of associated work skills is provided in Table 11-1 (Egan et al., 1984). Notice that many of these, such as ''checks own work'' and ''works alone without disruptions for specified periods with no contact from supervisor or teacher,'' are examples of behaviors that can be taught within the context of other curricular activities, perhaps even before the student reaches secondary school.

The behaviors listed in Table 11-1 comprise the essence of prevocational training, which can be further reinforced in actual job situations. From this list, it is apparent that many of those skills that are essential for job success are communications skills or important behavioral or social skills that should be routinely taught in the school. These skills are an essential part of students' instructional programs and should be included in their Individual Education Programs (IEPs) (see Chapter 10), even in the early intervention years. As will be shown, these skills are also an essential component of the vocational training program.

For some time, teenagers and adults with Down syndrome have participated in work activities in segregated settings, usually called *sheltered workshops* or *work activity centers*, which provided supervised, usually routine work at a slow pace. It is now known that people with Down syndrome can be trained on the job for employment in ordinary jobs in the community.

Zucker and Altman (1973) described an on-the-job training program for adolescents who were mentally retarded. They reported the placement of two of the graduating students into full-time employment; after 1 year, both students retained their positions. Then the literature became silent on the topic of community-based job training for adolescents until 1979. During that year, Becker, Wildener, and Soforenko (1979) presented the positive forecast that opportunities were expanding for community-based competitive employment. In that same year, Adams, Strain, Salzberg, and Levy (1979) reported on a model program that included on-the-job training for adolescents who were moderately and severely handicapped.

The terms *chronological-age-appropriate* and *functional* curriculum became part of the lexicon for secondary programs with an article by Brown et al. (1980). Many people inferred from those terms that vocational training would be community-based. Yet there are few examples of

Table 11-1.
Associated Work Skills

Work-related behavior

    Checks own work

    Corrects mistakes

    Works alone without disruptions for specified periods with no contact from supervisor/
        teacher

    Works continuously at a job station for specified amount of time

    Safety

        Uses appropriate safety gear

        Responds appropriately during fire drill

        Follows safety procedures specific to classroom/shop

        Wears safe work clothing

        Cleans work area

        Identifies and avoids dangerous areas

        Responds appropriately to emergency situation (sickness, injury, etc.)

    Participates in work environment for specified periods of time

    Works in group situation without being distracted

    Works faster when asked to do so

    Completes work by specified time

    Time management

        Comes to class/work for designated number of times per week

        Recognizes appropriate time to take break or lunch

        Recognizes appropriate time to change task

    Observes classroom/shop rules

    Does not leave work station without permission

Mobility and transportation

    Takes appropriate transportation to and from school/work

    Locates work station/desk

    Locates bathroom

    Locates break/lunch area

    Locates locker or coat area

    Moves about class/work environment independently

Self-help grooming

    Dresses appropriately for school/work

    Cleans self before coming to school/work

    Cleans self after using restroom

    Cleans self after eating

    Shaves regularly

    Keeps hair combed

    Keeps nails clean

    Keeps teeth clean

    Uses deodorant

    Bathes regularly

Cares for menstrual needs
Cares for toileting needs
Eats lunch and takes break
Washes before eating
Brings lunch/snack independently
Operates vending machine
Uses napkin independently
Displays appropriate table manners

Social communication

Communicates basic needs
Thirst
Hunger
Sickness
Toileting needs
Does not engage in
Self-stimulatory or self-abusive behavior
Aggressive/destructive behavior
Self-indulgent (attention-getting) behavior
Engages in relevant, appropriate conversation
Responds calmly to emotional outburst of others
Talks about personal problems at appropriate times
Refrains from exhibiting inappropriate emotions at school/work
Refrains from bringing inappropriate items to school/work
Refrains from tampering with or stealing other's property
Responds appropriately to changes in supervisors/teachers
Interacts with co-workers/students at appropriate times
Responds appropriately to social contacts such as "hello" or "good morning"
Initiates greetings appropriately
Ignores inappropriate behaviors/comments of coworkers/students
Refrains from inappropriate sexual activity at school/work
Laughs, jokes, and teases at appropriate times
Responds appropriately to strangers
Approaches supervisor/teacher appropriately when
Needs more work
Makes a mistake he/she cannot correct
Tools or materials are defective
Does not understand task
Task is finished
Disruption has occurred
Sick
Complies with supervisor/teacher's requests in specified period of time
Responds appropriately to correctional feedback from supervisor/teacher
Responds appropriately to changes in routine
Follows instructions

community-based vocational training conducted during school years. Alper (1981) presented systematic and replicable procedures for a community-based vocational training program. Firth and Edwards (1982) reported on a program in Calhoun, GA, that placed eight students with moderate retardation, aged 13–19, in competitive jobs. Wehman and Pentecost (1983) and Wehman, Kregerl, and Barcus (1985) described a complete model for placement of students with moderate and severe handicaps in competitive employment training and placement. None of these authors focused exclusively on youth with Down syndrome, yet we must infer that some students with that handicapping condition were included in the reported studies. This chapter includes some specific case histories of young people with Down syndrome to show their progress with competitive employment training.

IMPLEMENTATION OF VOCATIONAL TRAINING

The program described in this chapter has been successfully implemented in four communities in Oregon with populations of 2,500, 12,000, 25,000, and 45,000. Across the four communities, more than 80 students each year are placed in competitive or supported jobs in the community (as opposed to sheltered workshop placement). These students range in handicapping conditions from mild to severe and have a wide range of disability conditions, some of which are Down syndrome.

The overall plan for each student is to begin vocational training at the middle school or junior high school level or when the student is in the seventh or eighth grade. Until students reach high school, they are placed in vocational settings for about 5-6 hours a week. These settings include motels, restaurants, plumbing shops, animal hospitals, universities, hospitals, supermarkets, and a variety of small businesses. During the first 3 years of high school, the time is increased to approximately 10 hours a week. During this time, all vocational placements are made in nonpaid positions and, as a result, there is more freedom to move students from one position to another. Once a student is paid, the focus is on the obligation to the employer instead of on the education and training of the student.

The general plan is that a student will have two or three placements a year. Normally, students will have mastered a job in 4 months. To expand the students' experiences and skills, they are then moved to another vocational setting or assigned to do a job with more complexity within the same vocational setting. Occasionally, students are retained in one job location but are given a wide variety of experiences in that one location. For instance, one young man with Down syndrome worked in a carpenter shop. His initial duties were to clean the shop. He then progressed to cutting kindling, which the carpenter sold. Finally he was employed making frames and boxes.

PAID EMPLOYMENT

When a student is within 18 months of graduation, paid employment is sought, and the goal is to have the student graduate while holding at least two part-time jobs. This concept does not preclude the idea of full-time placement but the placement in part-time jobs has many advantages, as summarized below.

Part-time jobs ranging in time from 3 to 20 hours are plentiful even in communities with depressed economies (see Table 11-2 for a list of companies providing employment in one community). Some employers need extra help but do not want to become committed to hiring another full-time employee; thus, a part-time employee is a welcome addition. However, many employers also recognize that part-time employees usually have a high turnover rate, leaving jobs after only a few months of employment. Thus, having the additional help with a reduced potential for high turnover due to the support of the training personnel is a pleasant prospect for an employer. Occasionally, employers need assistance to identify part-time job opportunities in their workplace. The vocational coordinator and job coaches have assisted many employers in the identification and development of those part-time positions.

Many of the jobs that are available to workers with more severe handicaps are boring because they are repetitive tasks that are not too complex and that are performed all day long. If a worker performs two or three different repetitive jobs during the day, boredom is significantly reduced. Also, by moving among a number of jobs, the employee has the opportunity for more interactions with more nonhandicapped fellow workers. Moreover, movement between job sites frequently provides other opportunities for social contact such as on the bus or while walking.

There is one major disadvantage to placement in part-time jobs; the worker is not entitled to the fringe benefits that frequently come with full-time employment. However, if the worker is receiving Supplemental Security Income (SSI) payments and has Medicaid benefits, these benefits may not be essential.

VOCATIONAL TRAINING PROCEDURES

The first step in job training is to locate a job for the student. This is usually accomplished by the vocational coordinator for special-needs students or by job coaches, who frequently uncover jobs for students as

Table 11-2.
Places of Employment

Pepsi-Cola Bottling Company
Towne House Motel
Oregon State University
    Grounds maintenance
    Kitchen
    Personnel
    Veterinary medicine
    Forestry sciences laboratory
Anthony's Restaurant
Citizens' Bank
Boys and Girls Club
Vandehey's Cabinet Shop
North's Chuckwagon
Covallis Art Center
Cirello's Pizza
Bressler's Ice Cream Parlor
Beaver Plumbing
Vivian's Beauty Parlor
U-Haul
Benton County Fairgrounds
Ark Animal Hospital
West Hills Animal Hospital
Applegate Feed Store
Albertsons Food Market
Rogers Apparel
Avery Square Shopping Center
Forrest Bowman Rental Properties
La Cantina Restaurant
Burst's Candy Store
Fred Meyer Shopping Center
Lyon's Restaurant
Nendel's Motel
Philomath Fire Department
Fabricland

they move around the community. Since paid positions are not sought for the younger students, the employer is asked only to provide a work experience site. Moreover, the employer is guaranteed that the job will get done and that there will be a trainer available to conduct the training. Therefore, the employer has no commitment to either pay or training. Of course, many of these nonpaid positions later develop into paid positions as the employer sees the benefit of hiring a particular worker.

After the job has been located, the job coach who will be the student's trainer performs the job, writes a task analysis (Table 11-3), and then introduces the student to the job. The job coach models the job for the student, then asks the student to perform the job and records data on the form shown in Table 11-3. The example shown represents only one component of a job; each job may have a number of components. A detailed set of procedures is developed to provide appropriate cues, consequences, and data keeping in an unobtrusive manner at the job site. This set has been described by Fredericks et al. (1987).

The job coach remains with the student each day until the student begins to master the various components of the job. At that point, the job coach begins to fade out of the job, allowing the student to demonstrate more and more independence. This fading process is gradual so that the student remains confident that he or she can perform the tasks required. Most students can master most jobs within a 4-month period.

As a student is being trained in a job, it will become apparent that certain associated work skills must also be taught. These will be added to his or her program as needed. For instance, a student may have to learn how to check in and out using a time clock or may have to use public transportation to get to and from a job. These associated work skills are additional tasks to be taught.

There is also the issue of inappropriate behaviors. Failing to greet fellow workers, stopping work because of distractions in the work place, and slow performance are examples; many more are included in the list in Table 11-1. If these behaviors are present, they are systematically observed and a treatment program is designed to remedy them. A complete description of how to implement programs to remedy these behaviors is provided in Egan et al. (1984).

CONTINUED SCHOOL CONTACTS

While supporting the concept of community-based instruction, one must not overlook the need for quality interaction time with peers. These two curricular needs can pose an inherent tension in the scheduling of the student's program. At the secondary level, there are prime opportunities within the school day for interaction with peers without Down syndrome. These include lunch time, physical education classes, some social studies classes, home economics classes, and after-school activities. Therefore, when scheduling vocational training in the community, every effort should be made not to conflict with these opportunities for social interaction.

CASE HISTORIES

Each of the following people with Down syndrome was followed for 2 years in school. Their names have been changed to comply with confidentiality requirements. These case histories have been selected to

Table 11-3.

Example of a Task Analysis and Data Sheet

Program _____   Name _____
Terminal objective _____

1. Turns on dishwasher	x	x	x	x	x	x	x	x	x	x	x	x	x
2. Turns on garbage disposal	x	x	x	o	x	o	x	x	x	x	x	x	x
3. Turns on trough garbage disposal	x	x	x	x	x	x	x	x	x	x	x	x	x
4. Puts garbage in hole on left	x	x	x	x	x	x	x	x	x	x	x	x	x
5. Puts utensils in hole on right	x	x	x	x	x	x	x	x	x	x	x	x	x
6. Puts dishes in trough	x	x	x	x	x	x	x	x	x	x	x	x	x
7. Puts coffee cups in rack on top of shelf	o	o	x	x	o	x	o	x	x	x	x	x	x
8. Puts small glasses in rack on top	x	x	o	x	x	x	x	x	x	x	x	x	x
9. Puts dishwasher rack sideways in loading area	x	x	x	x	x	x	x	x	x	x	x	x	x
10. Puts bowls face down in dishwasher rack	o	o	o	o	x	o	x	x	x	x	x	x	x
11. Puts dishes upright in dishwasher rack	x	x	x	x	x	x	x	x	x	x	x	x	x
12. Puts trays upright in dishwasher rack	x	x	x	x	x	x	x	x	x	x	x	x	x
13. Puts ashtrays and large glasses face down	o	o	o	x	o	o	x	x	x	x	x	x	x
14. Pushes full rack into machine	x	x	x	x	x	x	x	x	x	x	x	x	x
15. Puts full coffee and glass rack in dishwasher	x	x	x	x	x	x	x	x	x	x	x	x	x
16. Drains utensils through utensil rack	o	o	o	x	o	x	x	x	x	x	x	x	x
17. Puts dishwasher utensil rack in dishwasher	o	o	o	x	o	x	x	x	x	x	x	x	x
18.													
19.													
20.													
21.													
22.													
Percentage of independence number of X's divided by the total number of steps.	71	71	71	94	76	93	94	100	100	100	100	100	100
Dates													
Trainer													

*Number of Xs divided by the total number of steps.

demonstrate a variety of situations and ages, and they are typical. The data presented are only a sample of the data available for each student but are representative of the data gathered for all such students with similar capabilities.

Case 1

John was a 17-year-old boy with Down syndrome in his junior year in school. His school placement was a resource room where he spent 3 hours a day. He was mainstreamed into other selected classes. He had no previous vocational training.

His initial placement in his junior year was in a cabinet shop where his job was to clean the shop. That job expanded within 30 days to the sawing of leftover scraps of wood so as to make kindling, which was bundled and sold by the shop. A sample of the data from this placement is provided in Table 11-4. There were four skill acquisition tasks to be taught. One associated work skill, working faster, was identified after the other skills were learned. Each of the skill acquisition tasks was task analyzed and broken into a series of smaller steps similar to the task analysis shown in Table 11-3. The percentages shown are the percentage of steps or the percentage of the total task that the student could perform independently. All of these skills were acquired within 2 months after the

Table 11-4.
Data for John at the Cabinet Shop

	Start Date	Data (%)*	Finish Date	Data (%)*
Skill acquisition tasks				
Sweeping/bagging sawdust: finish room	11/22	68	12/6	100
Sweeping/bagging sawdust: main shop	11/15	62	11/21	100
Starting work independently	12/2	50	12/9	100
Sawing kindling	12/5	83	12/13	100
Associated work skills				
Increase work rate: clean shop in 30 minutes	1/4	42.5 min	1/26	24 min

*Percentage of completed steps.

job commenced. The student stayed on this job for the remainder of the year. Because he was scheduled to graduate within 2 years, he was placed in a paid status after mastery of the job and was paid by the hour for the tasks described in Table 11-4. Toward the end of the school year and during the summer between his junior and senior year, he was given additional tasks to perform. He was taught to make boxes and frames and was paid by the pieces completed.

During John's senior year, another job was added when he was employed by an animal hospital. Table 11-5 provides the data for skill acquisition tasks and associated work skills for this job. One of the problems John had at this work site was his seeming unsociability. There were seven other workers at the site and he would not greet them when he came to work in the morning. When the trainer learned that John could not remember their names, John was rehearsed in the names with the use of Polaroid pictures of the employees. After that, John's daily greetings were much more consistent.

John was placed on the payroll at the animal hospital and worked there for the next 2 years. During his senior year, he was also placed on the payroll of the Fire Department at which time he quit his job at the cabinet shop. The Fire Department ran out of funds for the position 5 months later, and John was released from that job. He then was placed as a groundskeeper at a shopping mall.

Shortly after graduation from school, he moved into his own apartment with another handicapped youth. Because his apartment was in a neighboring town, he asked for assistance to find jobs in the town in which

Table 11-5.
Data for John at the Animal Hospital

	Start Date	Data (%)*	Finish Date	Data (%)*
Skill acquisition tasks				
Walking dogs	9/19	63	9/25	100
Cleaning kennels	9/19	64	10/1	100
Cleaning runs	9/19	94	9/26	100
Cleaning isolation kennels	9/19	94	9/26	100
Feeding animals	10/9	83	10/19	100
Associated work skills				
Clean kennels in an average of 6 minutes	10/26	7.7 min	11/15	5.28 min
Greet fellow workers appropriately	11/9	33	12/14	89

*Percentage of completed steps.

he was residing. (The groundskeeping job was located in that town.) He was soon placed as custodian for a day care program in a church. He now works at both the groundskeeping job and the custodial position. He works about 6 hours a day, including travel time between jobs, and earns approximately $240 a month. A third job is anticipated for him in the near future. He continues, of course, to receive his SSI payments in addition to his pay.

Case 2

Susan, who was 13-years-old and who has Down syndrome, entered the vocational program in eighth grade. The data for her job placements during that year are shown in Table 11-6. She had two placements during that year, each lasting slightly over an hour a day. The first was a grounds maintenance job at Oregon State University (OSU). She was trained there in a nonpaying job from the middle of November until the end of March in two skill acquisition programs and two associated work skills programs. In April she moved to the student cafeteria at OSU where she again worked slightly more than an hour a day. She stayed in that job until the end of the school year.

During her ninth-grade year, Susan was employed only for a little more than an hour a day and was still in unpaid job positions. During that year, she worked at the OSU veterinary medicine clinic where she folded

Table 11-6.
Data for Susan During the Eighth Grade

	Start Date	Data (%)*	Finish Date	Data (%)*
OSU grounds maintenance				
Skill acquisition tasks				
Grounds maintenance	11/16	69	12/6	100
Sweeping	1/4	50	1/17	100
Associated work skills				
Eye contact	2/1	38	3/30	85
On task	12/7	64.5 min	12/17	85
OSU kitchen				
Skill acquisition tasks				
Bussing tables	4/11	90	5/7	100
Loading dishwasher	5/4	33	5/21	100
Unloading dishwasher	4/17	62	4/25	100

*Percentage of completed steps.

surgical gowns and laundry for the operating room. In April she moved to Albertson's Food Market where she was given the job of caring for plants.

As Susan advances in school, she will be placed in more job experiences, two or three a year, until her junior year. At that time, the staff will confer with her, determine her job preferences, and try to locate appropriate paying jobs. Because Susan started in this program at an early school age, she will acquire a wide variety of job experiences and will be able to voice preferences based on reality.

Case 3

Noah, a young man with Down syndrome, was 19 years old and had never been in a vocational program. Noah also exhibited severe behavior problems. He ran away from school almost daily; at home he refused to get ready for school and would run away to avoid going to school. Every effort by parents and school to reinforce Noah for school attendance failed. Noah also exhibited other inappropriate behaviors. He walked in a style described by staff as "limbo," with his back arched backwards and his face lifted to the sky, a behavior that was certainly unsuited for any workplace. He also had difficulty completing tasks, and he was easily distracted.

At an IEP staffing, it was determined that Noah would continue to be enrolled in school since school attendance in the state for those with handicaps is permitted through age 21. However, Noah would not attend any classes in school but would be enrolled exclusively in a vocational program. Noah was initially placed in community vocational programs for 2 hours a day as a custodian in a youth center. This was a relatively isolated placement that allowed intensive one-on-one training with a trainer skilled in changing inappropriate behaviors. Within 3 months, the limbo behavior had disappeared, and Noah was independently starting his work and completing it on time. He then was placed in an additional nonpaid position washing U-Haul rental trucks. After training, he was able to perform that job independently. However, that job also presented little opportunity to interact either with other workers or with the general public. Therefore, during the second year, a plan was developed where Noah worked for 3 hours a day at the local work activity center and for 2 additional hours volunteered in a cooperative food store. Volunteering for otherwise paid positions for adults needs to be looked at critically to ensure that workers with handicaps are not being exploited. In this placement, however, which was in a cooperative establishment, volunteer workers are frequent, so Noah was doing no more than the other workers. The cooperative was a busy and distracting environment. It took Noah a few weeks to adjust to the extensive stimulation and distractions, but he now successfully performs his work tasks, such as marking prices on goods and placing them on the shelves. A job coach is still necessary but is now providing minimum direction and feedback.

The current plan for Noah is continued placement in both the activity center and the cooperative food store. Paid employment is now being sought and, at a later time, will probably substitute for the work time at the activity center.

OTHER FORMATS OF SUPPORTED WORK

This chapter has discussed supported work in the form of individual placement in the community. There are three other forms of supported work that should be considered, not only at the secondary level but also for adult placement.

The first of these is work on crews. For instance, a crew for adults has been established to perform garden and lawn care with individual contracts with homeowners or on an on-call basis. Apartment cleaning of vacated apartments for a property management corporation has required the establishment of a crew to perform the work. Crews usually consist of a job coach and three or four persons with handicaps.

Another form of supported work occurs in an enclave in an industry. In this arrangement, the industry assigns a body of work to be performed by a small group under the direction of a job coach. The enclave is an integral part of the industry, and the workers with handicaps have ample opportunity to mingle with the other workers.

Recently, a number of private businesses have been established by those with handicaps with support from job coaches. The most common of these is associated with the production of craft items that are then sold in fairs and street markets. Worker cafeterias in various businesses are run by people with handicaps, and there are greenhouses maintained by persons with handicaps who sell to the general public and to other nurseries.

AFTER GRADUATION

The individual placement model described herein leads to placement in jobs in the community upon graduation. Some form of competitive, supported work placement is ideal for an adult with Down syndrome. Unfortunately, the only vocational models available in most communities for the graduate are sheltered ones. Sheltered work was designed for those unable to work in the community. Persons with Down syndrome can

◆

successfully perform in a variety of competitive jobs in the community, and every effort should be made to achieve those types of placements. However, the workers need to be supported with a network of people to assist and ensure that these adults will be successful in their placements. Support for some can be a simple once-a-month check with employers to determine that all is going well. In other instances, support may be necessary every day.

Supportive services for competitive employment are not available to any significant degree in most communities. Parents and friends of those who have Down syndrome should actively lobby within their state governments, both at the legislative and executive levels, to establish on-the-job training and support services for residents with handicaps.

SUMMARY

Community-based competitive employment should be an integral part of the secondary level of public school for a person with Down syndrome. The model described in this chapter has been successfully implemented in four communities, and, at the time of this writing, an intensive training program is underway to train additional school districts in its use. Non-sheltered adult vocational programs are not available everywhere. Parent and professional groups can only make such services available by describing such services to political leaders and program administrators, and lobbying for establishment of such programs.

REFERENCES

Adams, T.W., Strain, P.S., Salzberg, L., & Levy, S. (1979). A model program for prevocational/vocational education with moderately and severely handicapped adolescents. *Journal of Special Education Technology, 111*(1), 36–42.

Alper, S. (1981). Utilizing community jobs in developing vocational curriculum for severely handicapped youth. *Education and Training of the Mentally Retarded, 16*(3), 217–221.

Becker, R.L., Wildener, Q., & Soforenko, A.Z. (1979). Career education for trainable mentally retarded youth. *Education and Training of the Mentally Retarded, 14*(2), 101–105.

Brown, L., Falvey, M., Vincent, L., Kaye, N., Johnson, F., Ferrara-Parrish, P., & Gruenewald, L. (1980). Strategies for generating comprehensive, longitudinal, and chronological-age-appropriate individualized education programs for adolescent and young-adult severely handicapped students. *Journal of Special Education, 14*(2), 199–215.

Egan, I., Fredericks, B., Peters, J., Hendrickson, K., Bunse, C., Toews, J., & Buckley, J. (1984). *Associated work skills: A manual*. Monmouth, OR: Teaching Research Publications.

Fredericks, B., Covey, C., Hendrickson, K., Deane, K., Schwindt, A., Perkins, S., & Gallagher, J. (1987). *High school vocational training for students with severe handicaps.* Monmouth, OR: Teaching Research Publications.

Firth, G.H., & Edwards, R. (1982). Competitive employment training for moderately retarded adolescents. *Education and Training of the Mentally Retarded, 17*(2), 149–153.

Wehman, P., Kregerl, J., & Barcus, J. (1985). From school to work: A vocational transition model for handicapped students. *Exceptional Children, 52*(1), 25–37.

Wehman, P., & Pentecost, J.H. (1983). Facilitating employment for moderately and severely handicapped youth. *Education and Treatment of Children, 6*(1), 69–80.

Zucker, S.H., & Altman, R. (1973). An on-the-job vocational training program for adolescent trainable retardates. *Training School Bulletin, 70*(2), 32–40.

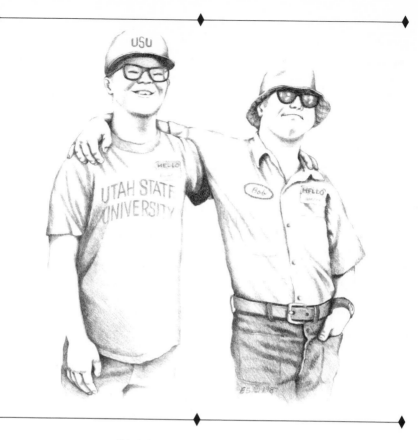

CHAPTER TWELVE

RECREATION: A PROMISING VEHICLE FOR PROMOTING THE COMMUNITY INTEGRATION OF YOUNG ADULTS WITH DOWN SYNDROME

JOHN E. RYNDERS AND
STUART J. SCHLEIEN

People with Down syndrome may not be inclined toward physical activity because of a tendency to have poor muscle tone and to be clumsy and overweight (Reid, 1985). They also, on the average, have lowered proficiency in both fine and gross motor abilities (Bruininks, 1974) (see Chapter 7). Couple their physical and motor limitations with communicative difficulties, such as problems with vocal expression and verbal learning (Rynders, Behlen, & Horrobin, 1979) (see Chapter 8)—abilities that are also frequently necessary in recreation programs—and it is easy to see why their participation rate is often low, not only in the school years but also in the adult years (Putnam, 1986; Putnam, Werder, & Schleien, 1985).

It might be tempting to suggest that the underutilization of recreation opportunities by people with Down syndrome is due to characteristics of Down syndrome; however, it is more likely that the low rate of community recreation participation, especially integrated recreation, is due to a lack of appropriate recreation opportunities. Ideally, these would involve nondisabled youths who have been prepared to interact with people who have Down syndrome in regular community activities. Successful community integration is a composite of what individuals with Down syndrome and nondisabled individuals contribute *mutually* to a recreation activity or to a relationship. Unfortunately, simply arranging for school-aged students with and without disabilities to be in physical proximity with one another does not, in and of itself, insure that positive interactions and interpersonal attraction will occur (Johnson & Johnson, 1975). Instead, accumulated evidence shows that without proper structuring of an interaction situation for mutually beneficial participation, nondisabled students often see peers with disabilities in negative and prejudiced ways (Jaffe, 1966; Novak, 1975), often feel discomfort and uncertainty in interacting with them (Jones, 1977; Siller & Chipman, 1967; Whiteman & Lukoff, 1964), and, during unstructured interactions, sometimes show feelings of rejection toward them (Goodman, Gottlieb, & Harrison, 1972; Iano, Ayers, Heller, McGettigan, & Walker, 1974). Thus, it has become clear that in order for positive attitudes toward people with disabilities to grow and thrive, information must be deliberately given to nondisabled people, and carefully structured integration experiences must be provided.

There is a tendency among many special educators and recreation personnel to invest a great deal of their energy and resources in segregated recreational programming. The intent and outcomes of programs such as

This work was supported in part by Contract No. 300-82-0363 awarded to the University of Minnesota from the Division of Innovation and Development, Special Education Programs, U.S. Department of Education. The opinions expressed herein do not necessarily reflect the position or policy of the U.S. Department of Education, and no official endorsement should be inferred.

the Special Olympics are laudable; however, they do not provide for all the recreational and social needs of people with Down syndrome because they are not designed to prepare peers with and without disabilities to interact with each other positively in integrated community settings.

PROMOTING INTEGRATED COMMUNITY RECREATION PROGRAMMING

Community volunteers such as 4-H club leaders can provide services to youths with Down syndrome by including them in the club with non-disabled members of a similar age. Special education teachers can help secondary school students with Down syndrome interact more frequently with age-matched nondisabled peers to prepare them for community life. Parents can encourage activity at the local YMCA for their adult child who never goes there because, "I don't know how to do anything there." In each of these situations, a comprehensive, step-by-step plan is very useful in facilitating appropriate participation and socialization. In conjunction with 5 years of studies in community leisure settings involving people with many types of disabilities, including Down syndrome, such a plan has been developed. Table 12–1 summarizes this four-part plan.

Table 12-1.
Conducting A Successful Integrated Community
Recreation Program for Youths with Down Syndrome

Stage A: Early Planning	Comments
Step 1: Clarify the integration motives and goals.	
First question: How can I help to insure that participants with Down syndrome *and* nondisabled participants benefit from the integrated experience?	Careful planning is necessary to have benefits for people with Down syndrome *and* people without disabilities.
Second question: Do I wish to focus on promoting social interactions? Recreation/leisure skills? Both social interactions and recreation/leisure skills?	Some activities have a rather low natural "valence" for promoting social interactions (e.g., painting a picture) while others (e.g., volleyball) are more oriented toward social interactions. Social interaction and skill development are combinable. Role of adult leader will change as a function of outcome decisions.

(continued)

Table 12-1 *(continued)*

Stage A: Early Planning	Comments
Third question: Do I want to create a peer tutor or peer friendship mode of interaction?	For peer tutor interaction mode, older nondisabled peers can be tutors. For peer friendship mode, same-age nondisabled peers can be friends. Both modes are legitimate; however, friendship mode emphasizes turn-taking, and cooperative interaction, and tends to be more fun. The peer tutor program tends to emphasize interactions that are more teacher-pupil oriented and that can become one-sided and less enjoyable.
Step 2: Think about practical matters.	
First question: How architecturally accessible is the program/facility?	If the space to be used is clearly marked and close to outside entrance, restroom, parking lot, and areas used by others, it will be more accessible for people with Down syndrome and others using the facility and will promote incidental integration.
Second question: How many people with Down syndrome can I handle, and how large should the integrated groups be that I construct?	Start slowly to be sure you are able to organize adequately a ratio of handicapped to nonhandicapped participants, e.g., 1 to 10, that is reasonably consistent with natural proportions of disabled to nondisabled in the general population.
Third question: What is the attitude of the potential nondisabled participants for integrated programming? How prepared are staff members in the recreation facility for integration in terms of their attitudes and training?	Don't *assume* that anyone is ready for integration. Prepare them *all* (see stage B for details about this preparation).
Fourth question: In terms of recreation activities themselves, are the activities	
Likely to be of interest to participants with Down syndrome and consistent with their educational and habilitation plans? Also of interest to nondisabled participants?	Activities should be chosen that will accommodate a wide range of interest and skill levels. Activities that are selected should always be chronologically age-appropriate and of interest to participants.

Stage A: Early Planning	Comments
Suitable for team, group, dyadic or solitary social activity? Appropriate for the simultaneous stimulation of skill development and social interaction?	Various activities emphasize differing interpersonal relationships. In planning it is necessary to make sure the person with Down syndrome has an opportunity to learn all the skills necessary to participate. For example, an adult leader might take an individual with Down syndrome aside (i.e., out of context) and teach him or her how to bait a fish hook before the person gets in the boat to fish with two nonhandicapped friends (in context).

Stage B: Advanced Planning	Comments
Step 1: Study the community recreation environment that you wish to involve.	
Identify particular challenges for the participants with Down syndrome in terms of special rules, procedures, equipment, and social and academic demands.	Contact the people who "hold the keys" to accessing environments, staff, and participants. Make detailed notes about all aspects of the environment, such as special rules, procedures, etc.
Discuss plans with the administrator of the program so that he/she becomes an advocate for integrated recreation programming. Keep in close contact as the program progresses so as to intensify initial support.	Some administrators may need to be "sold" on the idea to take full advantage of it.
Step 2: Increase the interest level of potential nonhandicapped participants in interacting with people who have Down syndrome.	
Show slides or a videotape of people with Down syndrome in integrated recreation settings.	A simple but very effective procedure is to take slides of potential participants with Down syndrome in the setting where integrated programming will occur. These can then be shown to nondisabled potential participants as a means of encouraging their participation.
Invite a person with Down syndrome to come and speak with the group about how he/she copes with activities of daily living, including recreation activities.	Choose a person with Down syndrome for this meeting whose language is intelligible.

(continued)

Table 12-1 *(continued)*

Stage B: Advanced Planning	Comments
Describe how a disability is a relative thing, i.e., it is something that all of us have in certain circumstances.	Nondisabled people must use a variety of tools and pieces of equipment to extend their strength, reach, vision, etc. In other words, having a disability is as much a matter of the demands of the environment as it is the capabilities of an individual. Part of this discussion should include the principle of partial participation. For example, if a bowling ball can not be rolled down the alley in the typical fashion, a bowling ramp or bowling ball pusher can be used to launch the ball.
Train a few adult volunteers to be able to encourage and reinforce positive peer interactions as they occur, and to provide advocacy and to "trouble-shoot" if required.	Social interactions do not always start spontaneously but need to be encouraged by adult volunteers and, then, reinforced in order to have them continue. Occasionally, a situation will need to be adapted or modified on-the-spot by the adult volunteer.
Step 3: Prepare a step-by-step description (task analysis) that specifies exactly what is to be done throughout every aspect of the program/facility/activity.	Often the task analysis takes the form of a comprehensive and highly detailed check list.
Modify the task analysis either to avoid problem areas or to overcome problems identified in the environmental analysis.	Avoid or element "trouble spots." For example, if an individual with Down syndrome is unable to speak clearly enough to order food items at McDonald's, he or she can be given small cards on which the desired items have been illustrated or written—either by the person with Down syndrome or by someone else.
Individualize the task analysis for each person with Down syndrome.	All individuals have different skills and problems. Modify according to physical, language, cognitive, and social abilities.
Step 4: Sharpen friendship skills of nonhandicapped participants by preparing them to interact cooperatively with peers who have Down syndrome.	The terms, *friendship* and *cooperative* are not synonymous but are highly interrelated. Although volunteers may be willing, they may lack experience interacting with individuals with Down syndrome and may have images of them that are unrealistic.
Sharpen awareness of what friends do as they interact (e.g., friends take turns, smile, stay close, make frequent eye contact, say nice things to each other, etc.)	We all from time to time could use such reminders.

Stage B: Advanced Planning	Comments
Give tips on how the nonhandicapped peers can help their friends with Down syndrome through difficult tasks without giving too much help.	Teach a hierarchy of helping prompts that begins with verbal instruction; then moves to demonstration and—if necessary—physical help along with verbal instruction. Emphasize that friends always keep a friendly voice and soft touch.
Provide instruction on how to communicate with a person who has Down syndrome, who may have expressive language difficulties.	Teaching nondisabled peers a few useful nonverbal signs can be interesting for them as well as increasing their motivation for communication—a fundamental part of friendship.

Stage C: Implementation	Comments
Step 1: Use the task analysis as a teaching guide, noting how successful each learner with Down syndrome is at every step of the recreation activity.	
For the initial presentation of the task, it is useful to offer each of the steps without doing any teaching, to see what the person already knows how to do.	On the task analysis form, pencil in a plus for each step of the task analysis performed without any instruction except some simple words such as "go ahead," "what comes next," etc. If this simple verbal prompt does not bring about the correct response, record a minus beside that particular step of the task analysis. Go through all of the steps in this manner, assisting the person to perform those steps that he or she is not able to do on his or her own.
Run through the set of steps with the learner who has Down syndrome, but this time provide *teaching* for each step not accomplished independently.	For each step of the task analysis, record what type of help was offered (i.e., verbal direction, then demonstration with verbal instruction, then physical prompting or full physical guidance with verbal instruction).
Make certain to positively reinforce the learner for each step of the task accomplished correctly.	Saying things such as "You sure are good at that game!" will be reinforcing to the learner, increasing his or her motivation to continue to do well.
Step 2: Structure the recreation context for cooperative, peer-to-peer interactions.	Cooperation and friendship go hand-in-hand, cooperation being one of the most important activators of friendship.

(continued)

Table 12-1 *(continued)*

Stage C: Implementation	Comments
Create a situation in which participation is reinforced so that the benefits of interacting cooperatively are maximized.	The completion of a task should be structured as a whole group enterprise, each individual contributing *something* and receiving a prize, even if the contributions are not equal.
Prompt the participants with and without disabilities to play or work together if social interactions are not occurring spontaneously.	Sometimes social interactions begin too slowly. If so, an adult volunteer can prompt the pair of friends, e.g., "Charlie, why don't you turn the pizza slowly while Debbie puts the pepperoni slices on it?"
Have adult volunteers compliment participants for positive interactions.	Rewarding words should not be given out indiscriminately but only immediately after the response desired.
Periodically, talk with nondisabled participants alone, reminding them of what their interaction role is.	Sometimes nondisabled peers will forget or become bored with their role as a facilitator and become too autocratic, too laissez-faire, or sometimes too absorbed in their own projects.

Stage D: Follow-Through	Comments
Step 1: Stay in contact with recreation professionals to see if the person with Down syndrome continues to engage in the community program, and also to encourage integrated programming as much as possible.	Integrated programming does not continue "automatically" and usually needs a continuing show of interest from the 4-H community volunteer, parent, or Girl Scout leader, etc.
Step 2: Maintain contact with participants who have Down syndrome and encourage their utilization of community recreation opportunities.	People with Down syndrome often become sedentary, spending too much time in front of the TV set. They will need *continuing* invitation and encouragement in order to keep participating at the bowling alley, park site, video arcade, roller skating rink, public library, etc.
Step 3: Stay in contact with participants who have Down syndrome and those who do not, with special attention to those who live in the same neighborhoods, go to the same schools, etc., providing continuing encouragement to maintain their friendships.	People with Down syndrome will have a continuing need to be "reconnected" both with peers who have Down syndrome as well as with nondisabled peers. Homogeneous and heterogeneous friendships are *both* important, and neither should be neglected. In fact, once school ends, friendships between people with Down syndrome may become especially important, particularly if they are working or residing in facilities where there are few nondisabled peers available.

Successful implementation of this plan requires that special attention be given to the two major components of the plan: task analysis and cooperative learning structuring, (Table 12-1, stage C). To further understand these two crucial components, it may be helpful to examine how the components were employed in two studies involving young adults with Down syndrome who participated in recreational bowling programs in their communities.

TASK ANALYSIS

Utilizing a task analysis that broke down the steps necessary to use a bowling facility in a competent and functional manner, Schleien, Certo, and Muccino (1984) taught Jeff, a nonverbal adolescent with Down syndrome, to use a community bowling facility independently. Jeff was taught to initiate and complete a bowling sequence on his own (i.e., secure a bowling lane, obtain bowling shoes, bowl, and pay), order a soft drink from a concession area, and purchase a snack from the vending machine in the bowling alley. Eventually, he was also taught how to walk from his group home to the bowling alley with a friend.

Teaching the full use of a bowling facility was based on information gathered through a systematic observation of the facility. This procedure, referred to as an environmental analysis inventory (Table 12-1, stage B), led to the construction of a task analysis (Table 12-1, stage B, step 3), which included several adaptations to help Jeff to overcome, or avoid, problematic aspects of using the bowling alley. For example, since Jeff had little functional language, he was taught to use a small file card on which printed phrases (e.g., "I would like to bowl"; My shoe size is a men's 3") informed the attendant of his needs. (For a more detailed explanation of the use of an environmental analysis inventory in recreation settings, refer to Certo and Schleien [1982] and Certo, Schleien, and Hunter [1983]).

Choosing an appropriate bowling ball was simplified by determining that Jeff had sufficient strength to use the heaviest ball available in the bowling facility. Thereafter, he was taught to select a ball into which his fingers could be easily inserted and removed, regardless of weight.

Another obstacle involved teaching Jeff the standard number of steps used to approach the foul line with the customary side-arm movement of the bowling ball as it is released. This complex skill posed a problem for Jeff, who had difficulties with dynamic balance and coordinated movement, as do many people with Down syndrome. To overcome this obstacle, he was taught to use a simplified style of bowling that involved walking up to the foul line without swinging the ball, then engaging the full side-arm swing and releasing the ball at the foul line. Although this is not the most popular style, it is used by some nondisabled bowlers, and it appeared to be appropriate for Jeff.

Currency and coin counting skills were simplified as follows. Just before Jeff entered the bowling facility he was given $2.50 (i.e., two dollar bills and two quarters), which he kept in his right pocket. He was taught to pay for his shoes with one of the dollar bills before the start of a game and to pay for the bowling game with the remaining change in his pocket. He then purchased a drink with the remaining dollar bill, and received $.35 in change, the exact amount needed to purchase a snack from the vending machine.

Training sessions usually occurred twice each week for 1.5–2 hours per session. To prepare for a session, Jeff's instructor, a therapeutic recreation specialist, would check to see which step of the task analysis (Table 12-1, stage C) was to be used in beginning the instruction, based on his prior achievement. The following is an actual portion of Jeff's task analysis, the part that deals with shoe rental and requesting a bowling lane (Table 12-2).

To initiate a training trial within the task analysis shown in Table 12-2, the instructor gave a step-specific verbal cue (e.g., "Jeff, go to the bowling shoe counter"), reinforcing an appropriate response if one occurred. If the correct response did not occur, the instructor repeated the verbal cue and modeled the desired behavior. If the correct response was still not produced, the verbal cue was again repeated, and Jeff was physically

Table 12-2.

A Portion of Jeff's Task Analysis for One Component of Bowling Alley Use

---

Bowling

A. Shoe rental and lane requesting

　1. Enter through main entrance

　2. Proceed to control desk

　3. Inform attendant of interest to bowl by pointing at score sheet

　4. Take off street shoe (right or left) and place on counter (shoe is used as collateral)

　5. Communicate bowling shoe size by handing attendant a prewritten "shoe size" card; Jeff must hand card to attendant with no more than two requests from attendant for shoe size

　6. Pay for shoe rental by placing one dollar on counter top

　7. Take shoe size card and change from dollar and place in pocket

　8. Take bowling shoes and score sheet (with lane number written in corner) from counter top

---

From Schleien, Certo, & Muccino, 1984.

Following (A) shoe rental and lane request would come (B) bowling preparation, (C) bowling, and (D) postgame activity, for a grand total of 32 steps.

prompted (helped to move through or toward) the desired goal. Positive reinforcement was always offered following a correct response (Table 12–1, stage C, step 1).

Following the day's instruction, Jeff's instructor gave him a general verbal cue (e.g., ''Jeff, let's go bowling'') and recorded his performance on the steps of the task analysis. The instructor recorded, on the task analysis form, a plus for a step performed independently and a minus for a step not performed independently or performed inadequately.

Jeff acquired the three sets of skills (bowling, purchasing a drink, and use of a vending machine) in 30, 10, and 18 instructional sessions, respectively. At this rate, an adult volunteer could train an individual of Jeff's ability level in the combined set of skills needed for the complete independent use of a bowling center in just 6 weeks, with three sessions per week, if the three skill areas were instructed concurrently.

Findings of the Schleien et al. (1984) study showed clearly that chronologically age-appropriate and functional recreational skills can be taught if broken into small steps and if the learner is prompted and systematically given reinforcement.

A second study showed that youths with Down syndrome enjoy interacting cooperatively with nondisabled youths as peers in recreation activities.

STRUCTURING COOPERATIVE LEARNING

Rynders, Johnson, Johnson, and Schmidt (1980) designed a study that, as did the Schleien et al. (1984) study, involved the use of a community recreation bowling facility. The purpose of this study was to explore the effects of structuring various types of social interactions between nondisabled adolescents and adolescents with Down syndrome. To achieve this purpose, interaction occurrences across three social interaction conditions (i.e., cooperative, competitive, and individualistic) over a 7-session, 8-week period were compared. Participants were 30 adolescents from three different public schools in Minneapolis, MN, 12 of whom had Down syndrome; the remaining 18 were nondisabled students. These 30 students (18 females and 12 males) were assigned randomly to one of three conditions (cooperative, competitive, or individualistic) so that six nondisabled students and four students with Down syndrome, and equal numbers of males and females, were in each condition.

In the cooperative learning condition (Table 12–1, stage C, step 2), students were preinstructed to maximize their group bowling score to meet a set criterion (improvement by 50 pins as a group) and were encouraged to interact as friends, i.e., to offer each other encouragement (e.g., verbal praise), reinforcement (e.g., a cheer), and assistance (e.g., help in handling a bowling ball). In the competitive condition, participants were told that their purpose was to bowl the best score—that is, to compete. In the individualistic condition, students were preinstructed to try to improve their scores by 10 pins, concentrating on bettering their own score and not worrying about other bowlers' scores. Basic bowling instruction, identical for all three conditions, was given equally in all conditions throughout the 8-week study.

Using a frame-by-frame recording sheet, trained observers (two for each condition) categorized all intelligible verbal interactions between individual bowlers in each condition on a continuous basis.

Results showed that the number of positive heterogeneous interactions, that is, interactions in which adolescents with Down syndrome talked positively to nonhandicapped peers, or vice versa, was significantly higher in the cooperative condition than in either the competitive or individualistic conditions. In fact, the number of positive heterogeneous interactions in the cooperative condition was nearly eight times greater than in either the competitive or individualistic condition (see Table 12–3).

Furthermore, the relatively high level of positive heterogeneous interactions in the cooperative condition did not prevent relatively high levels of positive homogeneous interactions, i.e., interactions between people with Down syndrome or between those without. To the contrary, the entire positive social interaction network increased substantially in the cooperative condition, that is, students received more positive interactions both with similar (homogeneous) peers as well as across nonsimilar (heterogeneous) peers. This duality is an important finding, since it is desirable for people with Down syndrome to interact positively and reciprocally with other people who have Down syndrome, as well as positively and reciprocally with nonhandicapped people, since they will probably live, work, and enjoy leisure in both homogeneous and heterogeneous settings.

With regard to the effects of cooperative interactions on attitude and bowling scores, nondisabled students in the cooperative condition rated peers with Down syndrome in their group significantly higher than nondisabled students rated their peers with Down syndrome in either the competitive or individualistic conditions. Bowling scores were not significantly different across the three groups. This is, the type of social interaction structuring did not have a differential effect on bowling performance.

Possibly more revealing than the statistical results is what occurred in the competitive and cooperative conditions when a participant with Down syndrome bowled either a strike (a rare occurrence) or a gutter ball (a frequent occurrence). In the group structured for competition, success was not rewarded. When a bowler with Down syndrome released the ball awkwardly, and the ball rolled down the alley slowly to the end of the

Table 12-3.

Frequency of Interactions Among All Subjects by Conditions

Condition	Positive Homogeneous	Positive Heterogeneous	Neutral Homogeneous	Neutral Heterogeneous	Negative Homogeneous	Negative Heterogeneous
Cooperative	685	804	32	66	3	4
Competitive	200	69	29	7	12	5
Individualistic	444	103	37	26	19	19

From Rynders, Johnson, Johnson, & Schmidt, 1980.

alley, the group reacted with silence if the ball, miraculously, knocked down all of the pins. No word of encouragement was given. The competitive structure gives emphasis to "beating" everyone else. Therefore, a strike, by comparison, lowers every other bowler's score.

In the cooperative group, when a gutter ball was thrown by a bowler with Down syndrome, other bowlers often offered words of encouragement. Proper cooperative structuring creates a more accepting social atmosphere.

PREPARING ADULTS WITH DOWN SYNDROME

Adults as well as adolescents with Down syndrome can be prepared for community transition through training in the functional use of community recreation facilities. Although there are few adult education programs designed to teach independent life skills to people with Down syndrome, such training has proven beneficial.

Schleien and Larson (1986) prepared two adults with Down syndrome (one 27 and the other 29 years of age), both of whom had relatively low IQs (33 and 23, respectively, on the Stanford-Binet intelligence test), to use an integrated community recreation center near the group home in which they resided. Neither of the men had ever used the recreation center, even though it was located only six blocks from their group home.

Objectives of the study were to teach the two men, Charles and Lawrence, to walk together independently to the recreation center, to select and use effectively an age-appropriate activity/game in the center, and to generalize acquired skills to another community recreation center in the city.

Prior to the program, an environmental analysis inventory (Table 12–1, stage B, step 1) was conducted to identify the skills and procedures needed for an adult to participate independently in the center and with nonhandicapped peers. From the environmental analysis, task analyses (Table 12–1, stage B, steps 1 and 3) for three activities were constructed, involving (a) going independently to the center; (b) borrowing fooseball equipment, playing the game appropriately and returning equipment afterwards; and (c) returning independently to their group home.

Both Charles and Lawrence had limited expressive language and manifested social behaviors that were not conducive to adult-like functional independence. Moreover, their repertoire of recreational abilities at the outset of the program was not chronologically age-appropriate. For example, during their initial visit to the community recreation center, when the instructor offered the verbal cue, "use the recreation center," to see what they could do without training, Charles and Lawrence proceeded immediately to a nearby children's play area and played with children's toys.

After trying several tasks without instruction, training began using a cue hierarchy, error correction procedure (Table 12–1, stage C, step 1). For example, a verbal cue was given (i.e., "Charles, release the fooseball onto the table"), and social reinforcement (e.g., pat on the back, verbal praise) was provided by the instructor for a correct response. Within a 20-week period, all three recreational skills were mastered by both participants.

When the men were given an opportunity to use the skills in three different community centers in the city, they were able to perform the skills to 100 percent correct criterion in all but one trial. (The skill of walking to the recreation center independently could not be tested at the other three centers because they were not within walking distance of the group home.)

Seven months after the training, both men were able to perform 95–100 percent of the steps in all three skill areas without modeling, physical prompting, or social reinforcement.

More research is needed to know exactly how long individuals with Down syndrome can retain the skills without continual training. It is assumed that at least continued reinforcement will be necessary to maintain a functionally useful level of skill.

COMBINING TASK ANALYSIS WITH COOPERATIVE LEARNING

Don't these combinations of task analysis and cooperative learning create a paradox of sorts? Task analysis focuses on promoting an individual's functional independence; cooperative learning focuses on the individual's interdependent interactions within a group. Aren't interdependence and independence opposites? No. In fact, they can be highly compatible factors in integrated community recreation settings. For instance, if an individual with Down syndrome learns to use a bowling facility independently, he or she has learned to do things that groups do not ordinarily teach their members. And, conversely, success in cooperating interdependently within a group promotes independence, since positive reactions from a group of peers helps an individual to become more independent. Indeed, techniques of task analysis and cooperative learning have been combined successfully in experiments to train adults with other handicaps (Schleien, Rynders, & Mustonen, 1986; Vandercook, personal communication).

PRAGMATIC USE OF THE PRINCIPLES

Of practical importance to those interested in the lives of adolescents and adults with Down syndrome is the general application of successful management and training principles. This includes looking at desired skills not as one whole to be acquired, but as small individual skills to be mastered one at a time. Knowledge of the procedures can help the practitioner utilize resources to the best advantage by carefully assessing needs and teaching the most salient behaviors first. Once the major plan is devised, it may also be possible to teach volunteers to be trainers. Volunteers frequently try to help by performing the activity for the person rather than firmly but patiently expecting the person with Down syndrome to perform the task according to his or her skill level.

Understanding all of the variables in a situation may also help the practitioner become less discouraged and more patient; practitioners may learn to be pleased about small successes rather than expecting an entire program to be perfect.

CONTINUING EDUCATION IN THE COMMUNITY

The ability to learn to get along with other people begins, of course, in early childhood—but it also continues into adulthood. For adults with Down syndrome, a successful life in the community is only possible with the attainment of interpersonal skills that make their presence not only acceptable, but also enjoyable, to others. Members of public and professional communities talk and write more about children with Down syndrome than about adults with Down syndrome. One of the reasons this is true is that completely independent adult skills are frequently not developed by their early 20s in people with Down syndrome. Without training and assistance, the Jeffs, Charleses, and Lawrences must retreat during their adult years into segregated living arrangements and self-contained recreational activities. Surely the infant and child we have nurtured and trained is worth the effort of continued nurturance and training to maximize independence and social acceptance as an adult.

REFERENCES

Bruinicks, R.H. (1974). Physical and motor development of retarded persons. In N.R. Ellis (Ed.), *International review of research in mental retardation* (pp. 209–261). New York: Academic Press.

Certo, N., & Schleien, S. (1982). Individualized leisure instruction. In P. Verhoven, S. Shleien, & M. Bender (Eds.), *Leisure education and the handicapped individual: An ecological perspective* (pp. 121-153). Washington, DC: Institute for Career and Leisure Development.

Certo, N., Schleien, S., & Hunter, D. (1983). An ecological assessment inventory to facilitate community recreation participation by severely disabled individuals. *Therapeutic Recreation Journal, 17*(3), 29-38.

Goodman, H., Gottlieb, J., & Harrison, R. (1972). Social acceptance of EMRs integrated into a nongraded elementary school. *American Journal of Mental Deficiency, 76,* 412-417.

Iano, R., Ayers, D., Heller, H., McGettigan, J., & Walker, V. (1974). Sociometric status of retarded children in an integrated program. *Exceptional Children, 40,* 267-271.

Jaffe, J. (1966). Attitudes of adolescents toward mentally retarded. *American Journal of Mental Deficiency, 70,* 907-912.

Johnson, D.W., & Johnson, R. (1975). *Learning together and alone: Cooperation competition and individualization.* Englewood Cliffs, NJ: Prentice-Hall.

Johnson, R., Rynders, J., Johnson, D.W., Schmidt, B., & Haider, S. (1979). Producing positive interaction between handicapped and nonhandicapped teenagers through cooperative goal structuring: Implications for mainstreaming. *American Education Research Journal, 16,* 161-168.

Jones, O. (1977). Mother-child communication with prelinguistic Down's syndrome and normal infants. In H. R. Schaffer (Ed.), *Studies in mother-child interaction,* New York: Academic Press.

Novak, D. (1975). Children's responses to imaginary peers labeled as emotionally disturbed. *Psychology in the Schools, 12,* 103-106.

Putnam, J. (1986). Paper presented at the International Congress on Down Syndrome. Brighton, England: University of Sussex.

Putnam, J., Werder, J., & Schleien, S. (1985). Leisure and recreation services for handicapped persons. In K. Lakin & R. Bruininks (Eds.), *Strategies for achieving community integration of developmentally disabled citizens* (pp. 253-274). Baltimore: Brookes.

Reid, G. (1985). Physical activity programming. In D. Lane & B. Stratford (Eds.), *Current approaches to Down's syndrome* (pp. 219-241). London: Holt, Rinehart, & Winston.

Rynders, J.E., Behlen, K.L., & Horrobin, J.M. (1979). Performance characteristics of preschool Down's syndrome children receiving augmented or repetitive verbal instruction. *American Journal of Mental Deficiency, 84,* 67-73.

Rynders, J., Johnson, R., Johnson, D.W., & Schmidt, B. (1980). Effects of cooperative goal structuring in producing positive interaction between Down's syndrome and nonhandicapped teenagers: Implications for mainstreaming. *American Journal of Mental Deficiency, 85,* 268-273.

Schleien, S., Certo, N., & Muccino, A. (1984). Acquisition of leisure skills by a severely handicapped adolescent. *Education and Training of the Mentally Retarded, 19*(4), 297-305.

Schleien, S., & Larson, A. (1986). Adult leisure education for the independent use of a community recreation center. *Journal of the Association for Persons with Severe Handicaps, 11*(1), 39–44.

Schleien, S., Rynders, J., & Mustonen, T. (1986). *Using applied behavior analysis approaches to integrate children with severe handicaps into an outdoor education environment*. Minneapolis: Consortium Institute for the Education of Learners with Severe Handicaps at the University of Minnesota.

Siller, U., & Chipman, A. (1967). Attitudes of the nondisabled toward the physically disabled. New York: New York University.

Vandercook, T. (1987). Personal communication: Doctoral dissertation data. Minneapolis: University of Minnesota.

Voeltz, L. M. (1982). Effects of structured interactions with severely handicapped peers on children's attitudes. *American Journal of Mental Deficiency, 86,* 380–390.

Whiteman, M., & Lukoff, L. (1964). A factorial study of sighted people's attitudes toward blindness. *Journal of Social Psychology, 64,* 339–353.

APPENDIX

GROWTH CHARTS

GROWTH CHARTS FOR CHILDREN WITH DOWN SYNDROME
FROM BIRTH TO 36 MONTHS

These charts provide reference percentiles for children with Down syndrome from birth to 36 months of age. They are based on mixed longitudinal data for approximately 400 boys and 300 girls with Down syndrome born between 1960 and 1986 and reared at home. Children with congenital heart disease are included in the sample. The centile rank for a given child indicates the relative position he or she would hold in a series of 100 children of the same sex and age with Down syndrome. For example, a child at the 10th centile is larger than 10% and smaller than 90% of children of the same sex and age with Down syndrome. The 50th centile is the middle position, and equivalent to ''average'' height or weight for a child with Down syndrome.

These charts correct for both the smaller size and slower growth rate of children with Down syndrome, and a child with Down syndrome would be expected to conform better to centile channels on these charts than those on the NCHS charts. However, because deficiencies in growth velocity occur at varying time, and are of widely different magnitudes, a child may not remain in a single growth channel on this chart. Downward centile shifts are common between 6 and 36 months of age.

Children with moderate or severe heart disease show greater growth deficiencies than those without or with only mild heart disease during the first three years of life. On the average, boys with significant cardiac disease are 2 cm smaller, and girls are 1.5 cm smaller, than those without, or those with only mild disease beginning in the first six months of life. As with normal children with heart disease, catch-up growth may occur following surgical repair or spontaneous closure of the lesion.

Weight gain for children with Down syndrome is more rapid than height growth. This often results in excess weight by 36 months of age. The etiology of this problem is not well understood, but may relate to decreased activity level and/or appetite disorder. Because the present charts reflect this tendency toward excess weight, they should always be used in conjunction with charts for normal children when assessing body weight.

GIRLS WITH DOWN SYNDROME
PHYSICAL GROWTH
1 TO 36 MONTHS

NAME _____ RECORD#

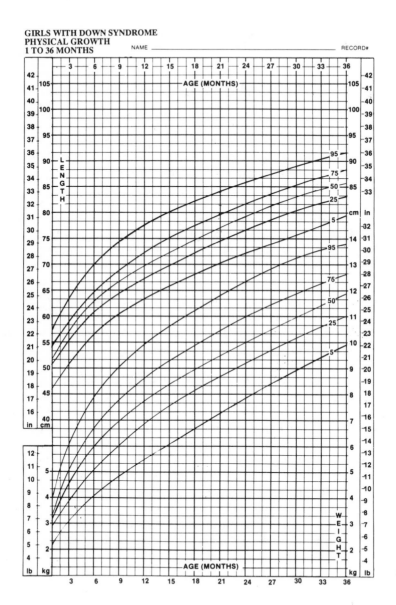

BOYS WITH DOWN SYNDROME
PHYSICAL GROWTH
1 TO 36 MONTHS NAME _____ RECORD#

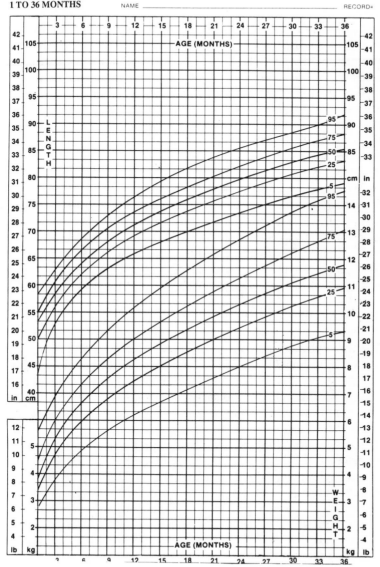

GROWTH CHARTS FOR CHILDREN WITH DOWN. SYNDROME FROM 2 TO 18 YEARSm

These charts provide reference percentiles for children with Down syndrome from 2 to 18 years of age. They are based on mixed longitudinal data for approximately 400 boys and 300 girls with Down syndrome born between 1960 and 1984 and reared at home. Children with congenital heart disease are included in the sample. The centile rank for a given child indicates the relative position he or she would hold in a series of 100 children of the same sex and age with Down syndrome. For example, a child at the 10th centile is larger than 10% and smaller than 90% of children of the same sex and age with Down syndrome. The 50th centile is the middle position, and equivalent to "average" height or weight for children with Down syndrome.

These charts correct for both the smaller size and slower growth rate of children with Down syndrome, and a child with Down syndrome would be expected to conform better to centile channels on these charts than those on the NCHS charts. During the childhood years, children with Down syndrome grow very similarly to normal children. However, at adolescence their growth spurts tend to occur slightly later than normal, and are not as dramatic as those seen in normal children. A small percentage of children with Down syndrome do not have an adolescent growth spurt.

Children with moderate or severe heart disease show greater growth deficiencies than those without or with only mild heart disease during the first three years of life. On the average, boys with significant cardiac disease are 2 cm smaller, and girls are 1.5 cm smaller, than those without, or with only mild disease beginning in the first six months of life, and continuing up through the adolescent period. As with normal children with heart disease, catch-up growth may occur following surgical repair or spontaneous closure of the lesion.

Weight gain for children with Down syndrome is more rapid than height growth. This often results in excess weight by 36 months of age, which is often enhanced during adolescence. The etiology of this problem is not well understood, but may relate to decreased activity level and/or appetite disorder. Because these charts reflect this tendency toward excess weight, particularly in values for the 90th and 95th centiles, they should always be used in conjunction with charts for normal children when assessing body weight.

GIRLS WITH DOWN SYNDROME
PHYSICAL GROWTH:
2 to 18 YEARS   NAME _____ RECORD# _____

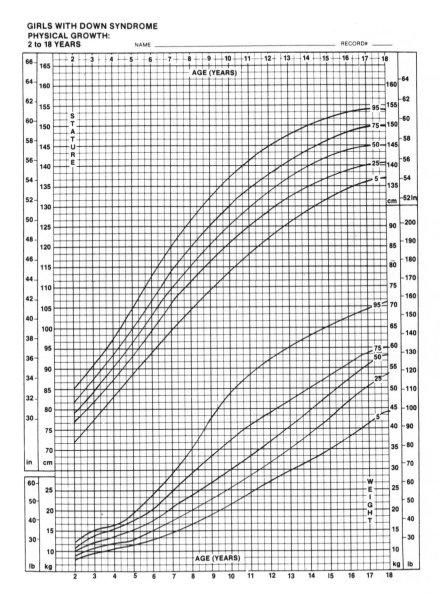

203

BOYS WITH DOWN SYNDROME
PHYSICAL GROWTH:
2 to 18 YEARS   NAME _____ RECORD# _____

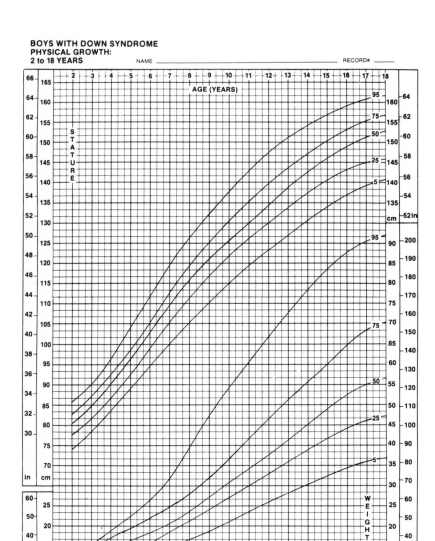

INDEX

Page numbers in italics refer to figures; those followed by a *t* indicate tables.

ISBN 0-316-84562-0

Also Available from College-Hill Press . . .

Communication Assessment and Intervention for Adults with Mental Retardation
Stephen M. Calculator and Jan L. Bedrosian

Pharmacotherapy and Mental Retardation
Kenneth D. Gadow and Alan D. Poling

Educating Disabled Persons for the 21st Century
Edward J. Cain, Jr. and Florence M. Taber

Effective Instruction for Special Education
Margo A. Mastropieri and Thomas E. Scruggs

Related Services for Handicapped Children
Morton M. Esterson and Linda F. Bluth

High-Risk Infants: Identification, Assessment, and Intervention
Louis Rossetti

Educating the Developmentally Disabled
Jan S. Handleman and Sandra L. Harris

Children on Medication, Volume One: Hyperactivity, Learning Disabilities, and Mental Retardation

Children on Medication, Volume Two: Epilepsy, Emotional Disturbance, and Adolescent Disorders
Kenneth D. Gadow

Genetics and Learning Disabilities
Shelly D. Smith

Birth Defects and Speech-Language Disorders
Shirley N. Sparks

Leisure Education for the Handicapped
Michael Bender, Steve A. Brannan, and Peter J. Verhoven

Sexuality and the Mentally Retarded
Rosalyn Kramer Monat